Medicare Made Easy 1999

Charles B. Inlander
President, People's Medical Society
and Michael A. Donio

MJF BOOKS

NEW YORK

The People's Medical Society is a nonprofit consumer health organization dedicated to the principles of better, more responsive and less expensive medical care. Organized in 1983, the People's Medical Society puts previously unavailable medical information into the hands of consumers so that they can make informed decisions about their own health care.

Membership in the People's Medical Society is $20 a year and includes a subscription to the *People's Medical Society Newsletter*. For information, write to the People's Medical Society, 452 Walnut Street, Allentown, PA, 18102, or call 610-770-1670.

Published by MJF Books
Fine Communications
Two Lincoln Square
60 West 66th Street
New York, NY 10023

Medicare Made Easy 1999
ISBN 1-56731-309-4

This edition published by arrangement with the People's Medical Society.

Manufactured in the United States of America on acid-free paper

MJF Books and the MJF colophon are trademarks of Fine Creative Media, Inc.

10 9 8 7 6 5 4 3 2 1

Contents

Acknowledgments

No book can be written by the authors alone. In this case, many hardworking and dedicated people assisted. We would like to thank the dedicated employees of the Health Care Financing Administration (HCFA), the people who administer the Medicare program. Especially we thank Carol Cronin, director, Center for Beneficiary Services; Elisabeth Handley, director, Partnership Development Group; Carole Sampson, Partnership Development Group; Anne Hoffnar, public affairs specialist with HCFA; Carter Warfield, Office of the Actuary; and many other fine people at the Baltimore headquarters who helped us launch this project.

We also thank Margaret Jefferson, health insurance specialist with HCFA, for her assistance on Social Security and Medicare eligibility criteria and Julie Walton, Medigap insurance specialist with HCFA.

From the People's Medical Society, we thank Janet Worsley Norwood, who managed the editorial revisions of this edition. We also thank Karen Kemmerer, who handled all aspects of production.

Introduction

Since 1983 when we created the People's Medical Society, I've traveled millions of miles listening and talking to people about medicine and health care. I've heard tales of horror and stories of inspiration. I've met victims of medical care and persons alive today because of it.

As a result of my travels, I have reached the following conclusions:

- Medical consumers want to be more involved in and in charge of their health care.

- People want reliable information about the quality of the services available so they can make informed medical decisions.

- Nobody can figure out Medicare!

About a month after the historic 1997 federal budget agreement, I saw the House Majority Leader conducting a town meeting in his Texas district. Among other things, he was explaining the changes the legislation had made in the Medicare program. As he went down the items, he stopped and said, "Frankly, I really don't understand much of this, but apparently people want it!" Aha!, I thought, if one of the architects of the Medicare changes cannot figure it out, nobody understands it.

Few government programs are in the news more than Medicare. It stands to reason. More than 39 million Americans are Medicare beneficiaries. So any changes or alterations in Medicare affect a lot of people. It is also the costliest government health program in the world. No national health program in any country spends more on its beneficiaries than Medicare does. That means legislators are constantly keeping an eye on expenditures.

Much has changed in the Medicare program over the past few years. The overall cost of the program has grown as the number of enrollees has increased. That, coupled with the high price of new medical technology and treatment, has put the long-term viability of the program under a cloud. And while the 1997 budget agreement keeps Medicare solvent into the next century, there is an ever-present concern that the program will be threatened when the baby boomers hit Medicare age.

But even bigger changes are coming as a result of the Balanced Budget Act of 1997. The Medicare+Choice program, which creates more options for beneficiaries, begins this year. So you have not only the option of the original Medicare program but also the option of a managed care plan, a private fee-for-service plan or a medical savings account. Sorting through these choices can be a daunting challenge. So we've added new material to help you analyze the programs and select the one that best meets your needs.

Over the past few years, the growth of Medicare health maintenance organizations has been phenomenal, and the number of beneficiaries selecting a Medicare+Choice managed care plan is expected to increase. More than 6 million people have joined them, with 100,000 more a month signing up. By 2005, it's estimated that half the Medicare beneficiaries will be in an HMO-type program. There have also been changes in what Medicare pays for and in what type of facilities the service must be performed. The fact is that Medicare rules, the services covered and the cost to consumers change every year. It is not easy to keep up with it all.

That's why we created *Medicare Made Easy*. This is the 10th edition of the book. It is the most comprehensive guide to Medicare published. And it is written directly for you, the health care consumer.

But why is there a need for a book like *Medicare Made Easy*? Doesn't the federal government publish booklets, brochures and pamphlets explaining the program? Why does a person need a book like this?

The government does, indeed, have some excellent publications explaining parts of the Medicare program. But they do not tell it all. They explain the basics, but they cannot give you hints and suggestions on how to get the most out of the program. And they do not publish it all in one place.

Medicare Made Easy has become the largest-selling book on Medicare because it is designed to empower the consumer. Each edition of the book is improved because of the feedback we receive from our readers. Plus, we are constantly watching the legislation and changes being made to the program. That guarantees you that the information found in these pages is the most up-to-date you will find.

In addition, *Medicare Made Easy* is written and published by the People's Medical Society, America's largest nonprofit consumer health advocacy organization. Our goal is to inform and assist you in getting the most from the health care system. We have no built-in conflict of interest—we do not sell health insurance or Medigap policies, we do not run health clinics or hospitals, and we are not doctors or other health professionals with an underlying agenda. We are *consumers*, just like you. And we are here to help you to become as savvy a medical consumer as you can be.

Medicare is not a charity program. You pay for it with premiums, deductibles and copayments. You elect the people to Congress who have the oversight responsibilities for the program. But it is not their program, it is yours! In our democracy, you are the chairperson of the board. Think of it that way when you use the services covered by Medicare. Demand accountability, respect and dignity from your health care providers. You deserve it.

CHARLES B. INLANDER
President
People's Medical Society
Allentown, Pennsylvania

Medicare Made Easy

Terms printed in boldface can be found in the glossary, beginning on page 239.

We have tried to use male and female pronouns in an egalitarian manner throughout the book. Any imbalance in usage has been in the interest of readability.

In this chapter you will learn: How Medicare began ▪ The role of the Social Security Administration ▪ The role of the Health Care Financing Administration ▪ The role of Medicare carriers and intermediaries ▪ The role of peer review organizations ▪ All about the Medicare+Choice Program

1. Understanding Medicare

Medicare is probably the largest and the most expensive single program run by the federal government. It is also one of the most complex because passage of the Medicare law in 1965 required a good deal of horse trading, especially with the **American Medical Association (AMA)** and various health insurers. If at times Medicare seems not to make sense to you, keep in mind that it's not supposed to. The current law is the result of a long series of political deals that had to satisfy diverse interests in order for there to be any law at all.

The Medicare program consists of two distinct parts: hospital insurance, or **Part A**, which provides payment for covered **inpatient hospital care**, posthospital extended care and home health care; and doctor insurance, or **Part B**, which helps pay for physicians' services, home health care services, hospital outpatient services and other medical services and items not covered under Part A. There is also a new part to Medicare called **Medicare Part C** or **Medicare+Choice**.

The Part A program is financed primarily through payroll taxes under the Federal Insurance Contributions Act (FICA). You've probably seen these letters on the stubs from your payroll checks. The Part B program is financed through a combination of general revenues and monthly premiums paid by each Medicare beneficiary. This premium is deducted from your Social Security check unless you specifically don't apply for Medicare Part B.

You won't think too much about Medicare until you need medical care. Assume that your health problems are simple and uncomplicated. Assume that all the care you need is within the bounds of what the program pays for. Assume that you have enough income to easily pay the Medicare Part B premium and the premium for a good supplemental policy. Assume that you have selected a good Medicare supplemental insurance policy. Assume that everything each of your doctors does is clearly medically necessary. Assume that you get well or die quickly. If all these assumptions are met, Medicare will appear benign and friendly. You will wonder why anyone ever has problems with it.

However, if Medicare is your only source of payment for health care, if you can't afford supplemental insurance or pick a poor policy or if you require care in a nursing home, Medicare can cause you nightmares. You will wonder how anyone could have designed a monstrosity that does to people what Medicare may well do to you. What you know can determine what kind of experience you will have with Medicare.

We have tried to keep this book short, simple and to the point. Our goal is to put you in the driver's seat when you, as a Medicare beneficiary, deal with doctors, hospitals, the assorted Medicare **carriers** and **intermediaries** and the large amount of paperwork involved. When we depart from the goal of KISS—keep it short and simple—it is to provide you with the background that you need to deal effectively with Medicare.

Medicare has been reformed continuously and piecemeal since it began, with layers of controls being added atop one another. To avoid cluttering the text with definitions and footnotes that the subject seems to demand and to help you break the code language of Medicare and medicine, we've printed special words in **boldface** to indicate that they are defined in the glossary at the back of the book. Points that we want to emphasize are in *italics*.

The American health care system embodies even more deals among the various parties involved than Medicare itself. They aren't public deals. Those who pay for health care in both the private and public sectors still don't feel as involved as they would like to be. Patients, consumers of medical services—you—have been involved in an effective way only since the early 1980s, when really productive health care consumer organizations emerged.

The impetus for Medicare arose in the early 1960s as part of the wave of New Frontier and Great Society programs started by President John F.

Kennedy and continued by President Lyndon B. Johnson. A repeatedly quoted figure was that the elderly, at the time the law was passed, spent about 15 percent of their incomes on health care—a figure that was thought to be intolerable, as Senator Hubert Humphrey proclaimed with tears streaming down his face, arguing for passage of the law on the floor of the Senate. That was in 1965.

Yet today the elderly spend *more* than 15 percent of their incomes on health care, even with the aid of Medicare. Does this mean that Medicare is a failure? Not really, if we measure it by other standards: Without it, the elderly and the disabled would spend far more than 15 percent of their incomes on health care, many would have to do without it, and the American people would have even less control over doctors and hospitals than they do today. And Medicare has helped to establish the idea that those who pay the bills in health care should make at least some of the rules.

Medicare has established, through **peer review organizations (PROs)** and their predecessors, that the medical profession and the hospital industry really cannot be trusted to guarantee quality care on their own. PROs are groups of doctors who make judgments about the medical necessity of what Medicare pays for, but they do it under contract with Medicare and aim for prices and limits set by Medicare. They are constantly producing evidence that doctors need professional checkups as much as their patients need medical ones. (A list of PROs is provided in appendix D.)

The **Diagnosis-Related Groups (DRG) system**, which we explain later, has shown that hospitals can give adequate care even if they are not rewarded with an endless shower of money. But Medicare has *not* relieved the elderly of the burden of paying for health care. It has only lightened it—and the elderly are paying more now, as a percentage of income, than when the law was passed.

In addition, Medicare does not pay for some of the services you may need the most. A common misconception, for example, is that Medicare pays for nursing home care. This misconception may have tragic consequences. Medicare will pay if you need short-term care in a **skilled nursing facility** to recover further after a hospital stay, but it does not pay for other nursing home care. **Custodial care**—care that you need because you can no longer function with complete independence—is *not* covered.

Medicare requires cost-sharing for most services, which means that you are responsible for a portion of the payment to the **provider**. In this respect, Medicare resembles private insurance plans, which also impose cost-sharing. This is, in theory, a good idea. In practice, however, it has meant the loss of the original goals—somewhat equal access to health care and elimination of the threat of impoverishment because of illness—for many Americans. The amounts that you must pay for the Part B (doctor insurance) premiums, for hospital care and for doctors' services are raised automatically as the result of a formula, without regard for your ability to pay.

Medicare has established a national fee schedule for compensating doctors called the **Resource-Based Relative Value Scale (RBRVS)**. Every **procedure** performed by doctors (both **primary care physicians** and **specialists**) is assigned a five-digit code along with a weighted value determined by the RBRVS. Medicare calculates the fee according to a formula that considers the resources needed to deliver the service. This system not only makes Medicare fees more attractive to doctors, but it also enables Medicare to more effectively manage expenditures on physician services. Another benefit is that more doctors might be encouraged to accept **assignment**. Only in Massachusetts, Pennsylvania and Rhode Island are doctors required to accept what Medicare pays.

A national pay scale had once been nearly unthinkable, in part because doctors are not required to treat Medicare beneficiaries. Ensuring access to health care for older Americans without such a requirement is a chicken-and-egg problem. Older Americans need money to pay for health care. They also need doctors who will see them for the amounts that they can afford. Contrary to the image of the sainted doctor tending all the sick, the AMA has maintained in its recent codes of ethics that doctors have no obligation to treat any individual. (Stopping treatment against a patient's wishes, or "abandonment," is different, however, and is considered unethical—but watch how fast you get abandoned if you can't pay your bill.) The AMA lobbied hard to ensure that no provision requiring doctors to treat beneficiaries went into the Medicare bill.

However, this hasn't stopped physicians and other practitioners from treating Medicare beneficiaries and participating in the Medicare program. More than 80 percent of physicians and other limited-license practitioners participate in Medicare. As a result, approximately 90 percent of Medicare-allowed charges are now billed by participating providers, which include medical doctors (M.D.'s), osteopathic doctors (D.O.'s), chiropractors (D.C.'s), nurse practitioners (N.P.'s) and physical therapists (P.T.'s).

There are, of course, Medicare supplemental insurance plans that claim to cover the costs that Medicare doesn't cover. Some of them do a decent job, but others don't; nearly all of them fail to provide coverage for long-term care, which imposes the greatest risk of financial ruin on the elderly. (Relatively few of the elderly run up hospital bills that are enormous compared with others, and Medicare still picks up most of the tab for hospital stays of usual length. It is long-term care, which about 5 percent of the over-65 population are using at any one time, that poses the real financial threat.) In this book we show you how to pick an affordable Medicare supplemental plan that fits your needs.

Medicare—and medicine—involve many terms that compress lengthy concepts into one or two words (for example, "assignment," meaning "the doctor's agreeing to take what Medicare determines is the fair price, handling the paperwork with Medicare for the patient, getting a check for 80 percent of the price directly from Medicare and charging the patient or the patient's insurer only 20 percent," which is rather cumbersome). Others are just medical or bureaucratic jargon, having the effect of giving the laity less control over the process by introducing what can amount to the secret language of a club.

The Law

Who really runs Medicare? The answers may surprise you.

Medicare, as it currently exists, is a compromise between politicians' desire to provide what they thought was good-quality medical care to the elderly and their fear of what it would cost. It's a compromise between doctors and hospitals who fear loss of control over patients and medicine in general and their desire for federal dollars. It's a compromise between the public's notion that health care is a right and the reality that even the federal government cannot enforce such rights throughout 50 states, the District of Columbia, Puerto Rico and the last two remaining territories—Guam and the Virgin Islands. Add the desire of large health insurers such as Blue Cross and Blue Shield not to be locked out of the picture. Like the camel, Medicare is a horse put together by a committee. And **Medicaid**—another federal health insurance program primarily for the nonelderly poor, which even the most starry-eyed legislators had not expected to see passed—was tacked on to the Medicare legislation at the last second.

Like other benefits provided by the federal government to the middle class, the current form of Medicare has become something of a sacred cow. Legislators and the public fear changing it because they fear losing what has been gained.

This means that in contrast to some other federal programs, much of the driving force for change comes from the small professional bureaucracy that runs the program and from the small segments of the other parts of government and the public that have learned to deal with that bureaucracy. Some of them toil on the staffs of congressional committees. Some work in the domestic policy section of the **Office of Management and Budget**. Others work in the **Congressional Budget Office**. Some are in universities. The inner workings of the Medicare program are almost as far removed from public scrutiny as those of the Department of Defense.

Congress could never adjourn if all the details of federal program management were worked out on the floor of the House and Senate. Laws passed by Congress broadly authorize the programs; appropriations passed as part of the federal budget each year provide money for them. Everything else is left to the various **executive departments**, which write regulations for them that "have the force of law." This means that they are just like laws passed by Congress, but Congress never passed them, and most members of Congress never see them. Except in very special situations, all of them are published in the *Federal Register* before they take effect. Just try finding the *Federal Register* at your local newsstand someday.

There's nothing sinister about this. It's a necessary compromise needed to make democracy work in a complicated society with thousands of government programs, a $1 trillion budget and only 535 representatives and senators to look after the whole thing. But it does mean that Medicare beneficiaries have to enter the fray along with the doctors, the hospitals, the insurers and all the other interest groups if they want their wishes to be heard, let alone heeded.

So here's who runs the parts of the show.

The Social Security Administration

The **Social Security Administration** is charged with determining who is eligible for Medicare. If you are applying on the basis of reaching age 65 and not on the basis of disability or **end-stage renal disease**, this almost always amounts to proving that you are who you say you are and that you were born when you say you were. If you are applying on the basis of disability, things usually get sticky (see chapters 2 and 8). The moment you are found eligible, your concerns with the Social Security Administration end. It passes on information to beneficiaries, and local offices act as a contact point for Medicare, but once the Social Security Administration has determined that you're eligible, you immediately become the responsibility of the **Health Care Financing Administration (HCFA)**.

The Health Care Financing Administration

HCFA was set up in the early days of the Carter administration to bring control of all federally funded health programs under one roof. (When we say "Medicare" in this book, we mean HCFA and the Medicare program as run by it.) The idea was that a single administrative agency would oversee not only the funding of these programs but also the services provided. What happened in practice is that a lot of public servants who had been under different roofs were lodged under one roof. Medicare and Medicaid have shared good ideas and come to resemble each other a lot more than they once did, but nothing miraculous has happened, except for the DRG system, which represents a major loss of power by the medical profession and hospitals and a major gain for the government. It is a model for moving the health care system away from professional interests and toward public interests.

Medicare controls every aspect of what happens to you as a Medicare recipient from the moment you are determined eligible. You are not handed back to the Social Security Administration until you die, at which time the Social Security Administration makes the determination on survivors' benefits.

HCFA has traditionally been charged with controlling the cost of medical care. In the course of trying to do that, it realized that Medicare and Medicaid laws only *seemed* to leave a lot of decisions in the hands of the carriers and the medical profession. Medicare has begun to assert control in almost every area, including many that doctors and hospitals and even the Food and Drug Administration, another part of the federal government, consider their own. For instance, Medicare has decided to release figures on the death rates and readmission rates for patients in hospitals around the nation. It is safe to say that as pressure to reduce the federal deficit mounts, Medicare will discover more things in the law that it has the power to do. Again, there's nothing sinister about this. Medicare always had the power to do much of what has been done by regulation. It has always had the power to find the prices charged by some doctors "inherently unreasonable" and refuse to pay them. Only recently has it found the will to do so.

HCFA can usually be counted on to try to do the right thing. But the medical profession and health care providers still retain enormous power in political circles, even if that power has diminished in recent years. The mood in Congress, the pressure to control health care costs and the activism of groups such as the **People's Medical Society** and the **American Association of Retired Persons (AARP)** created a climate in which HCFA can be used as a lever to expand the power of consumers in the health care system. This situation is not guaranteed to last, and Medicare has to be watched. You can deal with it in two ways: first, as a member of an association that asserts the rights of Medicare beneficiaries, and second, as an individual beneficiary.

What HCFA cannot do on its own, Congress has often been willing to do. Congressional committee staffers and the civil servants in HCFA talk with each other, and ideas are passed around. Regulations that Medicare does not have the power to issue tend to become laws in the very next Congress.

It is not editorializing, but just pointing out a fact, to say that this situation has come about because the hospitals and organized medicine have deeply offended some powerful congresspersons and senators in the past few years. Health care is so complicated that congresspersons who take the time to educate themselves about it are routinely deferred to by their colleagues. The current discord between Congress and organized medicine creates a great opportunity for the public to have a very loud voice in the way Medicare operates.

Carriers and Intermediaries

When the Medicare law was passed, health insurers demanded a role. Basically, they argued that Medicare would be socialized medicine and therefore unacceptable if the federal government ran it itself, but that it would be a boon to the public if the federal government gave them contracts to run it. They won, sort of.

Medicare contracts with health insurance organizations, called carriers and intermediaries, to process Medicare claims (intermediaries process Part A [hospital insurance] claims and carriers process Part B [doctor insurance] claims). A list of carriers and intermediaries for the various parts of the United States can be found in appendix A.

Medicare periodically holds competitions for the contract to be a Medicare carrier for a particular area. Those who want the contract write long, detailed proposals and submit them to Medicare. Medicare selects the one that looks like it can do the job at the lowest overall cost. Medicare then monitors the carrier's performance. The list of carriers and intermediaries in appendix A shows that the Blue Cross and Blue Shield plans were certainly not locked out as they had once feared.

The carriers and intermediaries try to implement the results of changes in the law and regulations according to manuals issued by Medicare. Sometimes they fail. The key to dealing with them is accurate paperwork and meticulous record-keeping.

Peer Review Organizations

PROs, as you may recall, are groups of doctors who make decisions on the **medical necessity** of health care under contract with Medicare. We explain how to deal with them in chapters 6 and 8. They are becoming an increasingly greater force within Medicare because HCFA relies on them for cost control.

The Medicare+Choice Program

Prior to passage of the **Balanced Budget Act of 1997 (BBA)**, Medicare beneficiaries had two options for coverage: the standard Medicare fee-for-service program or a **health maintenance organization (HMO)**. Medicare+Choice (pronounced "Medicare plus choice"), which came about as a result of the BBA, expands these options to include what are called **coordinated care plans: preferred provider organizations (PPOs)**, HMOs with a **point-of-service (POS)** option and **provider sponsored organizations (PSOs)**. The BBA also created **private fee-for-service plans (PFFSPs)** and **medical savings accounts (MSAs)**. Again, all of these fall under the heading of Medicare+Choice, which is sometimes referred to as Medicare Part C.

Don't let the alphabet soup frighten you. We show you how to sort through these options and pick the one that is best for you. *The bottom line is that you don't need to select a new plan if you're satisfied with your current Medicare coverage.* However, you may be able to obtain additional services (such as prescription drugs, hearing aids and routine dental care) through one of the new Medicare+Choice plans.

The creation of the Medicare+Choice program represents the most extensive overhaul of Medicare since it began in 1966, but only time will tell if these changes will improve the program as Congress intended.

How to Deal With All of the Above

In this section we discuss some points to remember in dealing with all of the above. We hope that things will go smoothly for you and that you will never have occasion to use your Medicare services.

The most fundamental point is that *Medicare is not a gift. You paid for it while you were working.* Medicare owes you services in the same way that a health insurer to whom you have paid premiums owes you services. In fact, you still pay a premium for Part B (doctor insurance). There is a contractual obligation to provide you with the services you've paid for, even if the federal government is the one with whom you have the contract.

Second, *being a Medicare beneficiary does not deprive you of any right you would have as a holder of private health insurance.* In fact, as you'll see in chapter 8, you have *more* rights than holders of private health insurance in all but a few states. Third, the price of health care has reached a level that very few individuals can afford. Most people are dependent on someone else—an employer, a parent or the government—for health insurance because health care has priced itself out of the private market. As far as health care is concerned, everyone is poor. Everyone needs help.

The Rest of the Book

This book has seven more chapters. Chapter 2 gives you an essential overview of the Medicare program and tells you how and when to apply. It also introduces you to the new Medicare+Choice options and explains how these plans are part of an expanded Medicare program. We provide worksheets so you can compare plans and select the one that best meets your needs. Chapter 3 details specific Medicare coverage under Parts A and B and also explains how services are covered, how they are paid and how the all-important "medical necessity determination" is made when care is required. Chapter 4 covers the very important issue of how to cover the gaps in Medicare with supplemental insurance. Chapter 5 explains how to make the most of your Part B coverage and why the **balance billing limits** will save you money. Chapter 6 explains your hospital coverage and how to ensure you get the care you need. Also covered is the appeals process. Chapter 7 covers nursing homes and **home health care**. Chapter 8 covers the problems that can arise and what you can do to solve them, as well as where to get help when you need it.

A final note: We believe that health care in one's later years should be a source of security and not one of endless worry. We hope that this book helps make it so.

In this chapter you will learn: How Social Security and Medicare are linked ▪ When you're eligible and how to apply ▪ How to overcome barriers and claim benefits ▪ How to file a claim for Social Security disability insurance ▪ What Medicare covers and what it doesn't ▪ Your Medicare+Choice options ▪ How to select a Medicare+Choice plan

2. The Basics

Many people are unaware of how relatively little of a person's necessary medical care Medicare covers. It's around 50 percent now, and that number is falling for many reasons. Medical care has become more expensive than Congress anticipated, and legislation is required to close the gap. At a time when federal deficits and the stability of the Medicare Trust Fund are major concerns, Congress is reluctant to increase benefits as long as beneficiaries continue to tolerate the situation. Doctors' fees have risen dramatically. Some of the nation's doctors still do not accept Medicare assignment for all patients, and Medicare has only recently begun to use its power to limit what it pays doctors. The combination of these factors drives up the doctor bill for both beneficiaries and the Medicare program.

This chapter deals, of necessity, with Social Security. Social Security and the Medicare program are entangled in the area of Medicare eligibility. Since we'll be talking about Social Security, it's worth noting that many people are unaware of how little of preretirement income Social Security is intended to replace—about 42 percent, on average. (The proportion falls as preretirement earnings rise. Lower-paid workers have a much higher replacement ratio than more highly paid ones.)

For both these reasons, it is important to know your Medicare and Social Security status before you retire. It is equally important to know what Medicare covers before you retire—possibly losing any coverage you might have through your employer—or before you drop any personal medical insurance coverage you might have.

Who May Apply for Medicare and Who Is Eligible

Anyone who thinks he is in one of the groups that Medicare covers can apply for it. In fact, if there is any doubt at all—in your mind or in the mind of the representative of Social Security at the **Social Security office** where you apply for Medicare—about whether you are eligible, you should apply.

The Basic Coverage Groups

Medicare was originally intended for "the elderly"—people 65 or older. It now also covers the following:

- Those who are **permanently and totally disabled**

- Those who have end-stage renal disease, the medical term for kidney disease that is severe enough to require **dialysis** or a transplant

Of course, things are not really this simple. Most, but not all, of the elderly are covered. The permanently and totally disabled are covered, but only if they meet the Social Security Administration's current definition of "permanently and totally disabled" and have received Social Security disability payments for at least two years. Those with end-stage renal disease are covered, but only if they have what meets the current definition of end-stage renal disease. For most people, becoming eligible is just a matter of turning 65 and applying. For a few, it can be a frustrating process involving lawyers, appeals and a lot of expense and anguish. What we try to do in this chapter is make the process as easy as possible for everyone involved.

Eligibility Requirements for Medicare Coverage

As mentioned earlier, Medicare is available to three basic groups of insured individuals—the aged, the disabled and those with end-stage renal disease. There are various eligibility requirements for each group.

To be eligible for Medicare, *you or your spouse must be entitled to payments under the Social Security Act or the Railroad Retirement Act.* This means, in general, that you must have worked for at least 10 years in a job that was covered under the Social Security Act or be covered *based on the **earnings record** of someone who is covered. You may also be eligible for Medicare if you a legal immigrant. (Legal immigrants are eligible only if they have resided in the United States for the past five consecutive years prior to application.)*

You must also be age 65 or older. If you are not yet 65, you may be eligible if you are permanently and totally disabled or if you have end-stage renal disease. A common misconception is that you will be covered if you are receiving Social Security. *This is not true unless you meet the requirements stated earlier.* The age requirements for Social Security and Medicare are different. For example, it is possible to start receiving Social Security payments at age 62, but you will not be covered by Medicare until you reach 65.

You are "eligible" for Medicare as soon as, and whenever, you meet the eligibility requirements that apply to you. You are "entitled" to Medicare only after you have *filed an application and are officially determined eligible. (If you are turned down, you have the right to appeal.)*

Work Requirement

In order to be eligible for Social Security and, subsequently, Medicare, you must earn a certain number of Social Security work credits called **quarters of coverage** and pay your Social Security taxes. One quarter of coverage is earned for every three months you work. While it may seem obvious, you earn quarters of coverage only when you are employed by a business that is covered under the Social Security Act. Fortunately, just about everyone, including the self-employed, are covered under Social Security. (Certain federal, state and local government employees pay only the Medicare portion of the Federal Insurance Contributions Act tax. In addition, some religious organizations are exempt from paying Social Security taxes. If you have any doubt as to your status, contact the Social Security Administration.) Most people pay the full Federal Insurance Contributions Act tax, so the credits they earn are usable to insure them for both Social Security and Medicare benefits.

In order for a quarter in which you work to count for Social Security (and Medicare) purposes, you must have a certain amount of income during the quarter. At present you earn one quarter of coverage for every

$700 in annual income. Therefore, if you make at least $2,800 during the year, you earn the maximum four quarters of coverage. *No more than four quarters of Social Security credit can be earned in any one year, regardless of your total income.*

This is very important because your eligibility for Social Security and Medicare is based on the number of quarters of coverage you've earned. Most people born after 1929 must earn 40 quarters of coverage (10 years of work) to be eligible for Social Security. This does not mean that you must work for 10 continuous years; rather, it means that you must accumulate 40 quarters of coverage during your working years. Even if you have gaps in your work record, you don't lose the credits you've earned. Let's look at the following example.

> *You work steadily for eight years and earn the maximum of 32 quarters of coverage; you then do not work again for three years. Since you were not working, you were not earning quarters of coverage during this three-year period. You then return to work and once again begin to earn quarters of coverage. Your count resumes at 32, and you eventually earn the 40 quarters of coverage needed for Social Security and Medicare eligibility.*

If you're like most people, you will earn more quarters of coverage than are required for Social Security eligibility. Earning additional quarters does not increase the monthly retirement benefit you receive (benefits are tied to your dollar earnings). A full discussion of your monthly benefit is beyond the scope of this book; however, we encourage you to use the form shown on page 31 to request a statement of your Social Security earnings and estimated future monthly benefit.

If you're not sure that you can qualify for Medicare on your work record and quarters of coverage, you may be eligible based on the earnings record of someone who is insured. For example:

- *Wives* are eligible if they are age 65 or older and if their husbands are insured.

- *Husbands* are eligible under the same conditions as wives.

- *Divorced women* are eligible if they were married to the insured person for at least 10 years, are age 65 or older and have not remarried.

- *Divorced men* are eligible under the same conditions as divorced women.

- *Widows and widowers* are eligible if they are 65 or older and were married for at least one year before the death of the insured spouse.

SOCIAL SECURITY ADMINISTRATION

Form Approved
OMB No. 0960-0466

☐ SP

Request for Earnings and Benefit Estimate Statement

To receive a free statement of your earnings covered by Social Security and your estimated future benefits, all you need to do is fill out this form. Please print or type your answers. When you have completed the form, fold it and mail it to us.

1. Name shown on your Social Security card:

First Name _____ Middle Initial ____

Last Name Only _____

2. Your Social Security number as shown on your card:

☐☐☐ — ☐☐ — ☐☐☐☐

3. Your date of birth

Month — Day — Year

4. Other Social Security numbers you have used:

☐☐☐ — ☐☐ — ☐☐☐☐
☐☐☐ — ☐☐ — ☐☐☐☐

5. Your sex: ☐ Male   ☐ Female

6. Other names you have used (including a maiden name): _____

7. Show your actual earnings for last year and your estimated earnings for this year. Include only wages and/or net self-employment income covered by Social Security.

   A. Last year's actual earnings: (Dollars Only)

   $ ☐☐☐,☐☐☐ . 0 0

   B. This year's estimated earnings: (Dollars Only)

   $ ☐☐☐,☐☐☐ . 0 0

8. Show the age at which you plan to retire:

   ☐☐ (Show only one age)

9. Below, show the average yearly amount you think you will earn between now and when you plan to retire. We will add your estimate of future earnings to those earnings already on our records to give you the best possible estimate.

   Enter a yearly average, not your total future lifetime earnings. Only show earnings covered by Social Security. Do not add cost-of-living, performance or scheduled pay increases or bonuses. The reason for this is that we estimate retirement benefits in today's dollars, but adjust them to account for average wage growth in the national economy.

   However, if you expect to earn significantly more or less in the future due to promotions, job changes, part-time work, or an absence from the work force, enter the amount in today's dollars that most closely reflects your future average yearly earnings.

   Most people should enter the same amount they are earning now (the amount in 7B).

   Future average yearly earnings: (Dollars Only)

   $ ☐☐☐,☐☐☐ . 0 0

10. Address where you want us to send the statement.

    Name _____

    Street Address (Include Apt. No., P.O. Box, or Rural Route) _____

    City _____ State ____ Zip Code _____

11. ☐ Please check this box if you want to get your statement in Spanish instead of English.

I am asking for information about my own Social Security record or the record of a person I am authorized to represent. I understand that if I deliberately request information under false pretenses I may be guilty of a federal crime and could be fined and/or imprisoned. I authorize you to use a contractor to send the statement of earnings and benefit estimates to the person named in item 10.

Please sign your name (Do not print)

▲

Signature _____

Date _____ (Area Code) Daytime Telephone No. _____

Form SSA-7004-SM (2-93) Destroy Prior Editions

- *Surviving parents* of a child eligible for Social Security benefits who were receiving at least half of their support from their child at the time of the child's death or disability are eligible at age 65.

These are the conditions under which most of us qualify for Social Security and Medicare. Medicare Part A begins the month in which you turn 65, provided you filed an application within the six prior months.

However, as mentioned earlier, there are two other ways to qualify: (1) if you are permanently and totally disabled (not able to work for 24 months) or (2) if you have end-stage renal disease and require dialysis (the mechanical filtering of blood) or a kidney transplant.

Qualifying for Social Security based on disability is not an easy task because what you might consider a disability isn't always a disability to the Social Security Administration. Under existing law, Social Security considers disability *your inability to work based on a medical condition. You will be considered disabled if you are unable to engage in any substantial gainful activity and only if your inability to work is also expected to last for at least a year or your disability is expected to result in your death.* Only the Social Security Administration can determine whether you are disabled based upon the information provided in your application for disability benefits.

The law requires that you have earned a certain number of quarters of coverage prior to your disability. The exact number of work credits you need for disability benefits depends on your age at the time you became disabled. Here's the formula for determining the quarters of coverage you need.

Disabled before age 24: You need six quarters in the three-year period ending when your disability began.

Age 24 to 31: You need credit for having worked half the time between age 21 and the time you became disabled. If you became disabled at age 29, you would need 16 quarters.

Age 31 or older: You generally need the same number of quarters as you need to be eligible for Social Security retirement benefits, and you must have earned at least 20 of the quarters in the 10 years prior to your becoming disabled.

Contact the Social Security Administration for information on the years of work credit and quarters of coverage needed for your specific age.

If you are disabled and entitled to Social Security or Railroad Retirement benefits, you are automatically entitled to Medicare Part A after 29 months.

To qualify for end-stage renal disease benefits, you must require regular dialysis or have had a kidney transplant.

In addition to having chronic renal failure, you must either be entitled to a monthly insurance benefit under Title II of the Social Security Act (or an annuity under the Railroad Retirement Act), be fully or currently insured under Social Security (railroad work may count) or be the spouse or dependent child of a person who meets one of the previous requirements.

Your first month of eligibility for Medicare Part A is the third month after the month in which a regular course of dialysis begins; however, this three-month waiting period can be waived if you participate in a course of self-dialysis training during the waiting period. If you receive a kidney transplant, your eligibility begins with the month of the transplant. It may begin up to two months earlier if you were hospitalized during this time in preparation for the transplant. For more information on the end-stage renal disease benefits program, contact the Social Security Administration and request HCFA publication No. 10128, *Medicare: Coverage of Kidney Dialysis and Transplant Services.*

Up to this point, our discussion has focused on the Social Security Administration and the role it has in determining your eligibility for benefits. Now we need to introduce you to another government agency and explain the role it plays in Medicare.

Until it is determined that you are eligible for Medicare, you are the responsibility of the Social Security Administration. Once you are eligible for Medicare, you deal with HCFA, which runs Medicare and Medicaid. (For the sake of brevity and avoidance of alphabet soup, we'll use "Medicare" to refer to HCFA from now on unless there's a clear need to distinguish the program from those who run it.) We'll discuss the application process later in this chapter. We are not trying to confuse Social Security issues with Medicare issues; until you are found eligible for Medicare, the two are tied together. Most of the advice we give on Medicare will also help you preserve or increase your Social Security benefits.

Entitlement and Enrollment Periods

We need to clarify the difference between when you are entitled to Medicare and when you may select or enroll in one of the Medicare+Choice plans. Once you meet the conditions for Medicare, age and quarters of social security coverage, you are entitled to enroll in the program. One of the following time frames should apply to you.

There are three types of entitlement and enrollment periods that apply to Medicare Parts A and B: the **initial enrollment period**, the **general enrollment period** and the **special enrollment period** for individuals who are still covered by an employer's health plan or disabled individuals covered under group plans. These enrollment periods *did not change* with the introduction of the Medicare+Choice program.

The initial enrollment period begins with the first day of the third month before the month in which you meet the Part A or Part B eligibility requirements. This period runs for a total of seven months. What this means is that you may apply three months before you meet the eligibility requirement, usually your 65th birthday, to three months past your 65th birthday.

The general enrollment period is much less complicated. It always occurs during the first three months of a calendar year: January, February and March. If you miss your initial enrollment period for any reason, you may apply during this general enrollment period.

You may delay signing up for Parts A and B and not pay a penalty for missing the initial enrollment period if you are still covered under your employer's group health plan. If you miss the initial enrollment period for this reason, you may apply during the special enrollment period, which begins on your 65th birthday and lasts for eight months or until you are no longer covered under your or your spouse's employer's group health plan. If you are disabled and covered under a group plan of a family member, the special enrollment period applies from the day you become disabled until eight months afterward or until you are no longer covered. (Contact the Social Security Administration to discuss your particular situation.)

Medicare is in the process of establishing uniform periods and methods for enrolling in and withdrawing from a Medicare+Choice plan. Once an **annual coordinated election period** is established, you will know when you can withdraw from a plan or select a different one. These changes are scheduled to be phased in until all Medicare beneficiaries, except those who are newly entitled, are on the same schedule.

We'll explain more on this later in this chapter.

What to Do If You Are Not Eligible Now

Remember: You cannot get Medicare unless you are eligible for Social Security. (There is an option to purchase Medicare as insurance if you're not eligible. We discuss this later.)

Two of the most common reasons you would not qualify for Social Security are (1) you aren't old enough or (2) you don't meet the work requirement. Only time will remedy these situations. (Remember: You can qualify for Social Security at 62, but you can't get Medicare until you are 65.)

If you are found ineligible because you do not have enough covered work, there's only one answer: earning the necessary quarters of coverage by working more.

Making Sure Your Earnings Record Is Accurate

You can obtain a statement of your earnings record every three years by completing Form 7004-SM from your local Social Security office (or by calling 800-772-1213) and sending it to the Social Security Administration. You can also send a letter. The letter below is a suggested format for this.

> Your name
> Your street address
> Your city, state and ZIP code
>
> Date *(Important!)*

Social Security Administration
Street address
City, state and ZIP code
ATTN: Proper person, if any

Dear Madam or Sir:

Please send me a copy of my earnings record. My Social Security number is *[fill in your number]*. My date of birth is *[fill in date]*. *[If you have used any other names]* I am also known as *[fill in the other names]*.

Thank you for your attention to this request.

> Sincerely yours,
> Your signature

If your earnings record does not show that you have enough covered quarters to be covered now, the first thing to do is make sure that the record is accurate. It can be in error about whether or not there were any earnings in a quarter. This can affect your eligibility for Social Security and Medicare. It can also be in error about the amount you earned. This can affect your eligibility for both programs and the amount of your Social Security benefits.

Errors in earnings records happen for a number of reasons. Failure of employers to report earnings to the Social Security Administration is probably the most common reason. To straighten out errors in an earnings record, the Social Security Administration has to check it against other records that are correct. This is where the hard part begins. Ideally, you will have all the paycheck stubs or pay envelopes that were ever issued to you, and you will have all of your federal, state and local tax returns for your entire working life. You will have the names and addresses of all your former employers. None of them will have shut down, moved or changed its name. If all this is true, straightening out your earnings record will be snap.

But as you can imagine, this is rarely the case. Fortunately, all you usually have to provide is information on the last five years of earnings, which are typically your highest-earning years (your Social Security payment is based on the "high five"). Those five years contain 20 of the 40 quarters you need to show that you worked, so all that is necessary is proving that you worked in 20 other quarters.

Personnel at your local Social Security office can help you straighten out your earnings record. The Social Security Administration has specialists in this at regional offices if the local office can't help you; your case can be sent to them as a last resort. The problem is that all of this will take time. For this reason, it is important to start early—before you need Medicare.

You may think you can see that your earnings record is right, but it's still a good idea to check it against your tax returns for the last five years of earnings. The figure recorded should equal the total of the Social Security Wages boxes on your W-2 forms. If you earned more than the maximum amount taxed for the year, only the maximum earnings for the year are shown. If more is shown, you can apply to the Internal Revenue Service (IRS), via an amended tax return for the years in which too much was collected, to get a refund of the excess. See the example on page 37.

Work and More Work

Another reason to check your earnings record is that you may not have worked long enough to receive benefits. Don't retire from your job assuming that you are eligible for Social Security benefits and Medicare. You may discover too late that you need additional quarters of coverage to qualify for Social Security benefits and Medicare. You may obtain a record of your earnings and your estimated monthly benefits by contacting the Social Security Administration (see page 35). Find out if you need more quarters of work in order to be covered.

This advice is obviously of no benefit if you have already quit and can't get your job (or any job) back or if you are permanently and totally disabled. We advise you to seek almost any sort of work you can do in order to obtain coverage. The benefits, perhaps although not as great as they should be, are well worth it.

Excess Social Security Taxes: Getting a Refund

In 1998, wages up to $68,400 were subject to a Social Security tax of 6.2 percent and a Medicare hospital tax of 1.45 percent, for a combined tax rate of 7.65 percent. Earnings above $68,400 were subject only to the Medicare hospital tax.

For example, by working two jobs, you earned $70,000. One paid $37,000, and the other paid $33,000. You did not reach $68,400 with either employer, so both continued to collect Social Security taxes.

You paid:	$37,000 × 7.65% = $2,830.50
	$33,000 × 7.65% = $2,524.50
	Total = $5,355.00
You should have paid:	$68,400 × 7.65% = $5,232.60
	$ 1,600 × 1.45% = $ 23.20
	Total = $5,255.80
Refund due:	$5,355.00 − 5,255.80 = $ 99.20

Applying for a refund of this amount will not reduce your future Social Security benefits because no more than $68,400 of income can be counted toward them.

Proving That You Really Are Disabled

If you believe you should be considered disabled, you should apply for disability benefits. The number of quarters necessary for coverage are reduced based on the year you became disabled.

You may be denied coverage if you do not qualify for Social Security benefits as a permanently and totally disabled person. Congress, in adding disabled person coverage, was acutely aware of the problems that had arisen in state workers' compensation programs and structured the law so that only unquestionably disabled persons would qualify. The definition used to accomplish this seems absurdly strict:

> *The term "disability" means (a) inability to engage in any substantial gainful activity by reason of any medically determined physical or mental impairment which can be expected to result in death or has lasted or can be expected to last for a continuous period of not less than 12 months, or (b) blindness; and the term "blindness" means central visual acuity of 20/200 or less in the better eye with the use of a correcting lens. (Social Security Act, Sec. 216[i][1])*

The regulations implementing the Social Security Act specifically prescribe that if you are able to perform any gainful work at all, you are not disabled for Social Security purposes. If the disability examiners judge that you could do some work, you are not considered disabled. You may protest that you do not know how to do the work the examiners believe you can do, that you have no chance of getting any training for it and that the only shop that does that kind of work is in Shanghai, but practical difficulties like this aren't considered—only your state of body and mind are. This definition leads to paradoxes: Persons likely to live a long time, but who are not "able-bodied" in any sense, are denied benefits.

There is obviously a large subjective component to an examiner's determination as to whether or not a person is disabled in the sense the Social Security Administration law requires. There is no exact medical standard that determines, for example, whether a person who has only partial use of one hand is capable or incapable of running a telephone answering service from home. The task is made harder because some disabled persons have achieved more than the vast majority of nondisabled persons: Some who have only the use of their eyes and mouth have written novels and painted; a quadriplegic who has lost the ability to speak but can still make sounds is one of the world's leading astrophysicists. Usually such individuals have an excellent social and financial support system (for buying special equipment and hiring assistants). Disabled persons who have this level of support and the drive to make use of it are rare. But the fact that they exist makes it easier for examiners to deny benefits to disabled applicants.

Sometimes examiners in the same office, to say nothing of examiners in different parts of the country, arrive at completely opposite judgments about whether or not specific persons meet the requirements for disability benefits. And politics seems to enter the picture as well. Some presidential administrations have placed great emphasis on strict applications of the rules; others have not. Courts in different **federal judi-**

cial districts have made different decisions about disability cases, and the **Department of Health and Human Services**, which includes the Social Security Administration and Medicare, is picking and choosing among these rulings in an effort to keep costs down. Your chance of being found eligible for benefits on the basis of disability depends, unfortunately, on the luck of the draw: what your doctor says, which examiner you get, the federal judicial district in which you live and which **administrative law judge** hears your appeal.

If you are denied benefits because you are found not disabled, we strongly urge you to appeal. But you should realize that time and costs will be involved and that you will probably need the help of a lawyer. We cover how to appeal decisions in chapter 8.

If You're Not Eligible, You Can Buy Medicare

Persons 65 years old or older who do not otherwise qualify for Medicare can purchase Medicare coverage just like private insurance. The 1999 premium for the combined Part A (hospital insurance) ($309) and Part B (doctor insurance) ($45.50) is $354.50 per month. Regulations permit those persons with at least 30 quarters of coverage to buy Part A at the reduced rate of $170 per month. Their Part B premium would be the same at $45.50 per month. Contact your Social Security office for more information about this program.

You are permitted to purchase Part B of Medicare (doctor insurance) if you are a resident of the United States, are 65 or over and are either a citizen or an alien lawfully admitted for permanent residence who has resided in the United States for the past five years. (It is under this rule that everyone enrolls in Part B.) If you are not eligible for Part A of Medicare, enrolling for Part B entitles you to purchase it, so you have to buy Part B to get Part A. For example:

Marge Smith, age 66, was married to her former husband, Harold, for nine years and 361 days. She would have been eligible for Medicare on his earnings record had she been married to him for 10 years. She is working and has earned 34 quarters of coverage, but she still needs 40 for full eligibility. She meets the age requirement (65 or over) and signs up to purchase Medicare. Because she has more than 30 quarters of coverage, she is able to purchase Medicare Part A at the reduced rate and Part B. When she is eligible, she will no longer need to pay the Part A premium but will still be responsible for the Part B premium.

How and When to Apply

Once more, being between ages 62 and 65 does not *entitle* you to Medicare. Being 65 or over does not *enroll* you for Medicare. It may take action on your part when you turn 65. Some people are automatically enrolled (this is called **automatic enrollment**); others are given notices that they need to enroll. Again, *if you want Medicare, apply for it.* The worst that can happen is that you'll find out your enrollment is already taken care of.

- If you are 65 or over and have been receiving Social Security benefits, you will automatically be enrolled for participation in Parts A and B. You will receive a notice and your card about three to four months before your 65th birthday. Your card will not be valid until you turn 65. You are covered for Medicare even if you do not have your card; the hospital can bill under your Social Security number even if you do not have the card. You can obtain a Temporary Notice of Medicare Eligibility from your Social Security office.

- If you are 65 or over when you apply for Social Security benefits, you will automatically be enrolled as part of the application process for Social Security. Your card will be automatically sent to you in the mail. You are covered for Medicare even if you do not have your card if you are over 65 and have been found eligible for Social Security benefits.

- Patients with end-stage renal disease are automatically enrolled if they are receiving Social Security disability benefits; otherwise, they must apply.

Your card also shows your health insurance claim number. Sometimes this claim number is referred to as your Medicare number. The claim number is your Social Security number followed by a letter. If an A and a B follow your Social Security number, you have both parts of Medicare. Your full claim number must always be included on all Medicare claims and correspondence. When a husband and wife both have Medicare, each will receive a separate card and claim number. Each spouse must use the exact name and claim number shown on his or her card.

It is important that you remember the following:

1. Always show your Medicare card when you receive services that Medicare can help you pay for.

2. Always write your health insurance claim number (including the letter) on any bills you send in and on any correspondence about

Medicare. Also, you should have your Medicare card available when you make a telephone inquiry.

3. Carry your card with you whenever you are away from home. If you ever lose it, immediately ask your Social Security office to get you a new one.

4. Use your Medicare card only after the effective date shown on it.

5. Never permit someone else to use your Medicare card.

You can apply for Part B Medicare coverage *to begin on your 65th birthday* anytime between three months before the month of your 65th birthday and the three months after. If you apply later than this, your Part A (hospital insurance) coverage will begin on the date you apply, not on your birthday. Your "personal enrollment period," as the Social Security Administration calls it, is these seven months.

Get It, Because You Can't Always Get What You Want

If you do not apply for Part B (doctor insurance) when you apply for Part A, you will not be eligible to apply until the next general enrollment period, which runs from January 1 to March 31 of each year. Your premium will be raised 10 percent for each year you wait to apply. In addition, your coverage will not begin until July 1 of the year you enroll.

We recommend that you apply for Part B coverage at the same time you apply for Part A, if you can afford it. Failure to take Part B will make any supplemental insurance you buy harder to obtain and will make your premium higher.

Low-Income Beneficiaries

Certain low-income Medicare beneficiaries may be eligible to have their state's Medicaid program pay for their Part B coverage. **Qualified Medicare beneficiaries (QMBs)** are eligible to have the state pay their Part B premiums and, in most cases, the deductibles and copayments.

In general, you must meet these eligibility requirements:

- You must be entitled to Medicare hospital insurance (Part A).

- Your monthly income must be at or below the federal poverty level for an individual or couple, and your resources may not exceed $6,000 (amounts are slightly higher in Alaska and Hawaii).

If you don't qualify for the Qualified Medicare Beneficiary program based on income, you may be eligible for assistance under the **Specified Low-Income Medicare Beneficiary (SLMB)** program. Individuals and couples are eligible for assistance if their incomes are up to 135 percent of the poverty level (amounts are slightly higher in Alaska and Hawaii). If you qualify, your state will pay your Medicare Part B premium, but not the deductibles and copayments. Contact your nearest welfare or Social Security office for more information.

The Specified Low-Income Medicare Beneficiary program has been expanded to provide some protection for those individuals with incomes between 135 percent and 175 percent of the federal poverty level. If you qualify, your state will cover the increase in the cost of your Part B premium that is attributed to the shift of home health care services. The state will not pay your entire Part B premium nor the deductible and copayments.

Application Forms and Process

Whether or not you are receiving Social Security benefits, you should apply for Medicare three months before your 65th birthday. This will allow ample time for all the paperwork to be processed and any questions about your eligibility to be answered so that you obtain coverage as soon as you are eligible.

The first step in applying for Medicare is to call your local Social Security office. These offices are commonly listed under the federal government section in the blue pages of your local phone directory. If you can't find a listing, call the information operator and ask for any Social Security office. Calling any Social Security office will enable you to find out which one you should contact.

Call that office. Tell them you want to apply for Medicare (and Social Security, if you are not already receiving it). The Social Security Administration is making a determined effort to carry out as much business as possible over the phone. This is generally more efficient, and it saves you a visit to the Social Security office. At the same time, if you have trouble dealing with matters like this over the phone (if, for example, you have trouble hearing and don't have an amplified phone), you can insist on a face-to-face visit.

Whichever way you apply, the Social Security office representative will fill out most of the forms for you. This is done to ensure that the type of answers the Social Security Administration needs to make a decision are obtained on the forms involved. After the representative has filled out the forms, you should read them—and insist on the correction of any errors—before you sign them. If you need special assistance (if, for example, you are deaf), special help will be made available to you. You may have to go to another Social Security office to find the right person to help you. The representative at the first Social Security office you go to will give you instructions. If you think you will need special help, you should mention this when you first call.

The representative will ask you to bring certain documents when you come to the Social Security office; usually, these include the following:

- Proof of age such as your birth certificate or a hospital birth record

- Records of earnings such as W-2 forms (or tax returns for the self-employed) for the past two years

- Your Social Security card

If you are applying because you think you should be considered disabled, you will be asked to bring some documents relating to your medical problems. The Social Security office representative will tell you what they are.

Keep your originals. Keep your originals. Keep your originals. Need we say more?

If you can't obtain your birth certificate or a hospital birth record, don't worry; the Social Security Administration also accepts the following:

- Census records

- Any school record that gives your age and was recorded before you were 21

- Newspaper birth announcements

- **Immigration and naturalization records**

- **Notarized affidavits** from people who are in a position to know your age

The Social Security Administration also accepts other types of proof.

There are three reasons for asking you to bring in proof of earnings. First, it lets the representative at the Social Security office determine quickly, between the earnings on your Social Security earnings record and the proofs of earnings that you bring in, whether or not you have the required quarters of coverage. If you're close, having this information when you apply can eliminate a lot of worry and another phone call or trip. Second, your Social Security benefits are supposed to be based on the highest five years of your earnings, and having current information avoids having to give you a smaller benefit now and a catch-up check and bigger benefits later, when the Social Security Administration computers get fed the information. Third, you may be receiving reduced Social Security benefits. Suppose you chose to retire at age 62, applied for reduced benefits and then took a job, or suppose you continued to work after 65 and earned enough to have your benefits reduced. In these cases, you are supposed to have your benefits recomputed periodically to take into account your additional earnings.

You also need not worry if you have lost your Social Security card. If you can remember the number, you can apply for a duplicate. If you can't remember the number, it is likely to be on other documents around your house, such as payroll stubs, credit card bills and insurance policies. If all else fails, the Social Security office can access its computer system, which will retrieve your name or any that sound like it. This considerably narrows the search for your number.

What Medicare Covers and What It Doesn't

A common misconception about Medicare is that it has a wide scope of coverage, comparable with the best private insurance plans. While it does cover hospital and physician services, there are limitations on days of care and rather large **copayments** if you encounter a lengthy hospital stay. In addition, there is no limit on your out-of-pocket expenses for services provided under Medicare Part B. Items such as hearing aids, eyeglasses, prescription drugs, dental care and custodial care are not covered.

The Meaning of "Coverage"

Coverage under Medicare is limited three ways, first by the services that are covered at all. By "covered" we mean that Medicare is willing to pay something for the service—not necessarily the full amount the provider wants, not necessarily enough to relieve you of all the burden of payment and not necessarily enough to attract enough providers to make the service routinely available, but something. (You may recall that a provider is a person or institution of a sort for whose services Medicare makes payments. Some providers are people; some are institutions such as hospitals.) Services for which Medicare will pay nothing are "not covered." The chart on pages 46-47 provides a brief summary of what is covered and what is not covered.

The Meaning of "Services"

Medicare covers "hospital services," but not all of them. Private rooms, **private duty nursing**, radios, televisions and telephones are among the services offered by hospitals, but Medicare does not automatically pay for them the way it does for, say, operating room charges. Medicare doesn't pay for private rooms unless they are prescribed by doctors or unless no other room is available. The same is true for private duty nursing. Radios, televisions and telephones are never covered. Medicare will not pay for the first three pints of blood used in blood transfusions in a year, but it will pay for all blood used after those first three. Any blood **deductible** paid under Part A or Part B applies, so you will have to pay for no more than three pints of blood in any year. The deductible is waived if you or someone else replaces the blood. Check with the local blood bank or the hospital blood bank on how to have a pint credited to your deductible.

Drugs administered in the hospital are normally covered, but those that have not been judged "safe and effective" by the Food and Drug Administration (FDA) are not covered.

All insurance plans have reserved the right, from their inception, to pay for what the carrier defines as covered, not anything a doctor may choose to prescribe or a patient may want. So, too, with Medicare. As the cost of medical care rises, limitations on payment by insurance companies and Medicare will increase, not decrease. Medicare and private insurers are likely to insist on more, rather than less, proof of safety and effectiveness before paying for a new service.

In the following sections, we discuss what is covered and what is not covered for each type of service. Chapter 3 explains how services are covered, when they are paid and the importance of a **medical necessity determination** when care is needed.

Hospital Services

Medicare covers the following services for inpatient hospital care:

- Semiprivate room (no more than two beds to a room)

- All meals, including any special diets that are needed, plus hyperalimentation

- Nursing services regularly provided by the unit you are in. (Medicare pays for nursing services in the **intensive care unit**, even though they are more expensive than those on the **general medical/ surgical floors**.)

continued on page 48

THE MEDICARE PROGRAM: WHAT IT PAYS, WHAT YOU PAY

Program services, as well as deductibles and copayments, are subject to change on a yearly basis. For the most current information, consult the latest edition of *Your Medicare Handbook,* available at most Social Security Administration offices.

Medicare Services	Benefit Period	Medicare Pays	You Pay
Part A: Hospital Insurance			

Hospital Services*
 Semiprivate room rate
 Miscellaneous hospital
   services & supplies
 Dietary & meal services
 Special care units
 Diagnostic procedures,
   x-rays, etc.
 Laboratory services
 Operating & recovery
   rooms
 Anesthesia & supplies
 Rehabilitation services
	First 60 days	All but deductible	Deductible of $768

	61 to 90 days	All but $192/day	$192/day
	91 to 150 days	All but $384/day	$384/day
	Beyond 150 days	Nothing	All costs
Skilled Nursing Facility Care In approved facility after a 3-day hospital stay and admitted to the facility within 30 days of discharge	First 20 days	All costs	Nothing
	21 to 100 days	All but $96/day	$96/day
	Beyond 100 days	Nothing	All costs
Home Health Care	Unlimited as medically necessary	All costs	Nothing
Hospice Care	Two 90-day periods One 30-day period	All costs but outpatient drugs and respite care	Limited drug costs and respite care
Blood Service	As medically necessary	All but the first three pints	First three pints

* Includes inpatient psychiatric care of 190 lifetime days.

Medicare Services	Benefit Period	Medicare Pays	You Pay
Part B: Doctor Insurance			
Physician & surgeon fees Therapists (physical/ speech/occupational) Diagnostic tests Medical supplies Ambulatory services Ambulance service	As medically necessary	80% of the approved amount after the $100 deductible	$100 deductible and 20% of the Medicare-approved charge (plus any cost above limited charges)
Outpatient Hospital Services	As medically necessary	Hospital costs	20% of hospital charges after the deductible
Home Health Care	As medically necessary	All costs	Nothing
Immunosuppressive Drugs	As medically necessary	One year of drugs used in immuno- suppressive therapy after transplant	Nothing
Blood Service	As medically necessary	80% of the cost after the first three pints	First three pints and 20% of cost

- Intensive care, intensive care units and care in other special care units (for example, a brain surgery unit)

- Drugs furnished in the hospital, unless they are excluded because the FDA has not found them "safe and effective"

- Blood transfusions, except for the cost of the first three pints of blood. (The cost of the blood can be met under the Part A [hospital insurance] or Part B [doctor insurance] deductible and will be waived if the blood is replaced.)

- Hospital charges for laboratory tests

- Hospital charges for x-rays and radiotherapy

- Medical supplies such as dressings, casts, splints, catheters and intravenous (IV) lines

- Use of **durable medical equipment** such as wheelchairs and crutches while in the hospital

- All hospital operating room and recovery room charges

- Rehabilitation services such as physical therapy and speech pathology provided during the **inpatient** stay

The charges of **hospital-based physicians** such as pathologists, radiologists, physiatrists and nuclear medicine and pulmonary specialists are not covered under Part A but are paid by Part B. This splitting of charges between the hospital and the physician for what looks like a hospital-provided service can often be confusing.

Medicare pays for a limited number of hospital days per **benefit period** (see pages 46-47) and has reinstated the spell-of-illness deductible. Each time you experience a spell of illness and are admitted to a hospital, you are responsible for the Part A hospital deductible. Remember: Medicare will pay only for services that are deemed medically necessary.

Before the enactment of the Diagnosis-Related Groups (DRG) system of prospective payment, limitations on days paid for by Medicare could have affected your hospital stay. The DRG system provides a set payment for each condition. In addition, there is a process that allows the hospital to apply for more money if your case is unusually expensive. Now you can be discharged only when hospital care is no longer medically necessary. The deal between the hospital and Medicare under the DRG system requires that the hospital provide as much service as Medicare patients' doctors deem necessary for their care.

You may think that Medicare pays for care anywhere in the world. It doesn't. Only care in hospitals in the 50 states and the District of Columbia, Puerto Rico and the last two U.S. territories—Guam and the Virgin Islands—is paid for. Care you receive in Europe, Canada, Mexico and the rest of the world is not covered. The only exception is if you are in the United States but are close to the Canadian or Mexican border and in need of emergency care, and the nearest hospital is in Canada or Mexico. In this situation, Medicare will pay for the services provided.

Another limitation on hospital services, mentioned briefly earlier, is medical necessity. We discuss this in more detail in chapter 6. For the moment, the general idea is this: Medicare will not pay for anything it does not consider dictated by the needs of good, professional medicine as applied to your case. Sometimes, for example in certain types of surgery that are often abused, the medical necessity determination is made before you go into the hospital or have the operation. In other instances, it is made after Medicare-mandated reviewers of coverage such as peer review organizations (PROs) review your chart and decide that your case has not been handled as it should have been. PROs control costs by monitoring services to determine if they are medically necessary and should, therefore, be paid for.

Medicare has been experimenting with ways to hold down costs ever since the program began to cost much more than anticipated in the late 1960s. PROs are one example of cost control in that they monitor the appropriateness of services to determine whether they are medically necessary and should be paid for. They are groups of doctors who contract with Medicare to make sure that the care given to Medicare beneficiaries is of acceptable quality and is really needed. The requirement that care be "reasonable and necessary" has always been in the law. PROs are just the latest means of enforcing it. They review some cases before care is given if local or national evidence indicates a high level of inappropriate use. In these situations, approval is required before Medicare pays. In other cases, they look at charts after the patient has been discharged and make decisions about the appropriateness of what was done. Finally, they review requests from hospitals for extra payment (over and above the amount the DRG system pays) and extra days of care.

Unless you have received an official notice that a service is not considered medically necessary before you have it done or that additional hospital days are not necessary before you decide to stay, you never have to pay for medically unnecessary care. We discuss in chapter 8 what to do when you receive such notices.

Physicians and
Related Services

Medicare pays for most services of physicians—holders of the degrees of Doctor of Medicine (M.D.) or Doctor of Osteopathy (D.O.)—and some of the services of podiatrists and chiropractors and dental surgery performed by dentists in a hospital. Some services of optometrists are covered as well.

Most **outpatient treatments** and tests such as electrocardiograms (EKGs), x-rays and physical therapy are covered. When the Medicare law was passed, most such services were performed in the **outpatient** departments of hospitals and were covered by Part A. Now most of them are available in physicians' offices and are covered by Part B, which means that they now require a copayment.

For coverage of nonhospital services (or Medicare services in general), the usual rule is that routine services such as annual physicals that are not aimed at treating a specific illness are not covered and that services designed to improve appearance or bodily function such as cosmetic surgery are not covered unless they are needed to restore a state of health that existed before illness or injury.

Outpatient psychiatric services are covered but require a 50 percent copayment. The limit on total lifetime inpatient psychiatric hospital days is 190 days.

At present, drugs and biologicals (hormones, serums, vaccines and such) are covered only if administered by the treating professional. They are not covered if they are prescribed for self-administration. Prescription drugs that the doctor prescribes for you to administer to yourself are generally not covered. The only exceptions are immuno-suppressive drugs such as cyclosporine, an antirejection drug prescribed for kidney transplant patients under the end-stage renal disease portion of Medicare.

Nursing Home
Services

Medicare coverage for a skilled nursing facility is limited to 100 days per benefit period, with full payment for the first 20 days and a copayment for days 21 through 100 (see page 46). *Medicare does not pay for nursing home care that is needed simply because you can no longer care for yourself.* The limited payment for skilled nursing facility services actually functions as a money-saver: If you need skilled nursing services to recover but can safely have them outside a hospital, it makes sense for the government to cover them in a lower-cost setting such as a nursing home.

The enormous expense of nursing home services—more than $70 billion annually—indicates that they have certainly helped many people who could not care for themselves. But the care given in many nursing homes is, frankly, of uncertain quality. Quality of nursing home care is not well monitored. Medicare has only recently decided to require that some sort of nurse (a registered nurse [R.N.], a licensed practical nurse [L.P.N.] or a licensed vocational nurse [L.V.N.]) be available on all shifts in all nursing homes. (See chapter 7 for more information on nursing home coverage.)

Other Services

Home Health Care: Home health care is covered for up to 21 consecutive days; there is no limit on the total number of visits. The major restriction is that the visits must be for medical care only. Homemaker-type services are not included. After 21 consecutive days, there must be a break of at least one day before another series will be paid for.

Flu Shots: Medicare covers the cost of flu shots. Also, an enhanced vaccine outreach program is available for beneficiaries.

Durable Medical Equipment: A number of pieces of durable medical equipment such as wheelchairs and hospital beds for home use are covered. If a doctor prescribes it, Medicare usually approves the equipment and pays 80 percent of the cost.

Products and Services for People With Diabetes: If therapeutic shoes are prescribed by a doctor, 80 percent of the cost is covered. Also, diabetes self-management training services, glucose monitors and test strips for people with type II diabetes are covered.

Eyeglasses, Contact Lenses and Hearing Aids: Eyeglasses, contact lenses and hearing aids are covered only if they are needed following eye or ear surgery or as a result of an eye or ear disease other than normal visual or hearing defects such as astigmatism, myopia and age-related hearing loss.

Medicare+Choice Options

When the Balanced Budget Act of 1997 was passed, it not only balanced the federal budget but also created the Medicare+Choice program (also called Medicare Part C), something that affects every Medicare beneficiary.

As a result, you can choose from a number of new health plan options in addition to the original Medicare program. We make this distinction between the original Medicare program (Parts A and B) and the new options because the Health Care Financing Administration (HCFA), the federal agency that runs Medicare, uses this language to identify the options available under the Medicare+Choice program.

Medicare+Choice options include the original fee-for-service Medicare program, **managed care plans** such as health maintenance organizations (HMOs), health maintenance organizations with point-of-service (POS) options, preferred provider organizations (PPOs), provider sponsored organizations (PSOs), private fee-for-service plans (PFFSPs) and medical savings accounts (MSAs).

In theory, these new programs give you the same marketplace health insurance choices enjoyed by those who are not in Medicare. Only time will tell if Congress did the right thing by creating these choices. However, we're going to do the right thing and tell you about your options and how to select the one that is best for you. Of course, the most important thing to remember is that *you don't need to make any changes if you are satisfied with your current Medicare coverage.* We can't stress this point enough. *You do not need to change your current Medicare coverage if you are satisfied.* We have also been assured that Medicare will stress this same point in all of its mailings to beneficiaries.

Availability of Medicare+Choice Options

Access to a Medicare+Choice plan depends on where you live and the types of plans available in your community. Although Congress intended to expand the choices available to Medicare beneficiaries, there's no regulation requiring such availability.

For example, managed care plans in your area may not have Medicare contracts or there may not be a provider sponsored organization in your community. Or a managed care plan may not offer a point-of-service option because it's too costly. A preferred provider organization might decide that contracting with Medicare is too complicated, leaving that option unavailable. Or perhaps none of the physicians in your community opts out of Medicare, and therefore there's no private fee-for-service plan available. Or maybe none of the insurance companies offers a catastrophic insurance plan that can be used in conjunction with a medical savings account.

For these reasons and others (for example, you may not be financially able to afford private contracting or you are physically unable to travel to different providers), your choices may be limited.

Medicare+Choice Election Periods

When the Medicare program consisted of Medicare Parts A and B or a managed care plan, you were permitted to enroll in or withdraw from a plan on a monthly basis. This current policy continues until the end of 2001. Beginning in 2002 and beyond, specific periods are designated as the **initial election period**, annual coordinated election period and the **special election period**.

If you've just become eligible for Medicare, your initial election period begins three months prior to when you are entitled to Medicare and ends the last day of the month preceding the month of entitlement. You will only have *one* initial election period. After that you are governed by the annual coordinated election period and the special election period.

The annual coordinated election period runs from October to December of each year. It's during this time that you may elect or select a different Medicare+Choice plan for the next year. Coverage in your new plan begins on January 1st of the next year.

There is also a special election period when you may change your Medicare+Choice plan due to circumstances beyond your control. Medicare defines these as when:

- Medicare terminates the contract of your Medicare+Choice plan.

- You are no longer eligible to remain in the plan you selected.

- You demonstrate to Medicare that your plan violated its contract by not providing the care you required in a timely manner, failed to deliver quality care or materially misrepresented itself.

- You meet such other exceptional conditions as determined by Medicare.

To complicate matters, a new policy is being phased in that affects current beneficiaries' rights to change from one Medicare+Choice plan to another. As you recall, the current month-to-month policy remains in effect until the end of 2001.

After 2002, if you first became eligible for Medicare prior to that year, you may change your Medicare+Choice plan once during the first six months of the year. You may go from original Medicare to a Medicare+Choice plan or from one Medicare+Choice to another, but only during the first six months of the year. If you first become eligible in 2002 or later, the guidelines of the initial election period that we describe earlier apply.

Beginning in the year 2003, your opportunity for changing from one Medicare+Choice plan to another or to original Medicare is limited to the first three months of the year. If you are unsure which period applies to you, contact the Medicare information line at 800-638-6833.

We begin by describing the types of managed care plans available under the Medicare+Choice program and then go into descriptions of the private fee-for-service plan and the medical savings account.

Types of Managed Care Plans

Managed care may be thought of as a combination of medical services and insurance in one integrated system that provides consumers with quality, cost-effective medical care. It is in essence a "hybrid" organization that determines how much medical care you need and how much it's willing to pay its providers for that care.

The basic idea behind managed care is that health care is less expensive if preventive services are covered and if there is no need for people to worry about the cost before seeking care. This makes sense. Managed care plans have clearly demonstrated that they can save at least 25 percent over the cost of care provided in a fee-for-service system (such as traditional Medicare), in which doctors are paid for each service they provide. It is thought that paying doctors for each service they provide gives them a perverse incentive to give care that is not really needed, and there is evidence to suggest that this is true.

Health Maintenance Organizations (HMOs)

There are four types of HMOs: group, individual practice association, network and staff.

In the group model, the HMO signs a contract with one or more large groups of physicians and hospitals to provide care to HMO members. These doctors are not salaried employees of the HMO but are employed by their groups. The doctors in these groups provide all of your medical care, and you must generally use them whenever you need medical services. However, some group HMOs are offering what is known as a point-of-service option. This permits members to go outside the group for care, although the group may impose additional fees.

An individual practice association is a type of HMO in which the plan's administrators sign contracts with large numbers of physicians—both solo practice doctors and doctors in group practices—to provide care to the HMO members. Physicians in an individual practice association agree to a negotiated set of fees paid by the plan.

A network model provides services through groups of doctors, hospitals and other health care providers who contract with managed care plans to care for consumers in the plan.

A staff model HMO employs doctors and other health care practitioners and pays them salaries. The doctors may also receive bonuses if the HMO does well financially. Typically, the staff model HMO owns the clinics and offices where consumers receive services.

All types of HMOs are available to Medicare beneficiaries. Medicare HMOs receive a set amount, based on the average cost of treating a Medicare beneficiary in the counties they serve, adjusted for local wage and price differences. For that fee they are required to provide all the services a Medicare beneficiary would receive in the traditional Medicare program, plus the deductibles and copayments. They may also offer additional services not covered under the traditional Medicare plan.

Health Maintenance Organizations with a Point-of-Service (POS) Option

Freedom of choice is a big issue with managed care plans because very often you are limited in your choice of doctors and hospitals and because you are required to use those doctors and hospitals when you need medical care. However, as a result of beneficiary complaints and a desire on the part of Medicare to make managed care more attractive, several options are now available to members of managed care plans with respect to provider choice.

Medicare permits what is called a point-of-service (POS) option. This means that you may choose providers who are not part of the managed care plan network and still have services covered. Selecting an out-of-network specialist, meaning one who is not part of the managed care network, is an example of using a POS option.

An HMO with a point-of-service option permits you to selectively go out of the network of providers to receive services. However, for this privilege, you are likely to have large out-of-pocket expenses in the form of deductibles and copayments.

Preferred Provider Organizations (PPOs)

PPOs are managed care plans with large networks of physicians, hospitals and other providers. They generally offer consumers a wider choice of doctors and hospitals than do HMOs. Usually, the benefits provided are significantly better if services are received from the preferred providers; however, for an extra fee, you can go to the doctor or hospital of your choice. On the other hand, you will probably be responsible for a deductible and copayment if you go outside the network of preferred providers. The extra cost can be trivial, or it can be so high that the PPO is, in effect, a managed care plan for all but the affluent. Generally, their benefits are not as generous as those of other managed care plans, but they are a little better than those of traditional fee-for-service plans.

Provider Sponsored Organizations (PSOs)

A PSO is a managed care plan owned by providers—either physicians or hospitals. These organizations won approval from Medicare to begin offering services to Medicare beneficiaries; however, because they are so new, no one knows exactly how they compare to other, more-established, managed care plans. Therefore, we can only suggest that you exercise caution and make sure you know how the plan operates before you join. Like all managed care plans, because PSOs are both insurance plans and medical plans, Medicare requires that they obtain a state insurance license before becoming eligible to compete for Medicare beneficiaries.

More About Managed Care

The type of contract the managed care plan has with Medicare affects the way in which you receive your services. There are two general types: risk and cost.

Risk-based plans have a "lock-in" requirement, which means that you *must* receive all covered services through the plan or through referrals made by the plan. With few exceptions, the only outside services covered are for medical emergencies. If you go outside the plan, you are responsible for all costs.

Cost-based plans do not have this lock-in requirement; instead, they permit you to use providers outside the plan; however, you are responsible for deductibles and copayments. In most instances the plan does not pay for services, but Medicare does. In this respect it's almost like traditional fee-for-service Medicare.

The Merits and Demerits of Managed Care

Some people do not like certain features of managed care plans, so managed care plans compete in other ways, often by offering more benefits than traditional insurance plans do. The same features that deter some people often attract other people. In some HMOs, for example, your choice of doctors is limited to those who are employees of the HMO (if it is a staff model HMO), to those who are in the group practices that the HMO has contracted with (if it is a group model HMO) or to doctors in private practice who have signed on as members of an individual practice association.

Opponents of HMOs make a big issue of the supposed denial of freedom of choice. It is little understood that Blue Shield, still the major supplier of insurance for doctors' services in the country, works on essentially the same principle: It will pay in full only for the services of doctors who are called Blue Shield-participating providers. The difference in HMOs is that no payment is made for services of any doctor not on the HMO panel unless an HMO doctor calls him in as a consultant or refers you to him.

Seeing a physician in a group or staff model HMO may be far more convenient for a person, especially a moderately sick one, than seeing a physician in private practice. Usually, primary care physicians (general practitioners, family practitioners, internists, pediatricians and obstetrician-gynecologists) are located in the same building with specialists. It may be possible to see a specialist immediately if the primary care physician thinks one is needed. **Outpatient surgery** suites, chemotherapy rooms, x-ray departments, laboratories and pharmacies are often located in the same building as the doctors' offices. HMOs pioneered "one-stop shopping" in medicine primarily as a means of cost control and as a convenience to their doctors, but it is a great convenience for patients as well. Some large HMOs even have their own emergency rooms located in their clinics.

Some, but not all, managed care plans try to make maximum use of physician extenders such as nurse practitioners, medical technicians and physicians' assistants. They do this based on research that shows that persons with these sorts of training can do as well as, or better than, doctors for a limited range of situations and can be trusted to recognize situations they can't handle and to call in the doctor. If you think of them as specialists in low-end routine care, you can be comforted by the evidence that they sometimes are better than M.D.'s. If your vision of proper medical care is having one specialist to look at your eyes, another to listen to your heart, a third to talk about your arthritis and a fourth to talk about your kidneys, a visit with the nurse practitioner will not make you happy. From the managed care plan's viewpoint, using physician extenders cuts costs, enables more people to be seen, gives them a sympathetic ear for problems to which the doctor seems too busy to listen and makes the best use of costly physicians' time.

Some managed care plans have a lot of general internists on staff and have **protocols** that require the other primary physicians to refer patients to them as special situations develop. This may lead to your switching doctors for no apparent reason while you are assured that there is no need to refer you to a specialist. Others treat internists as specialists in the use of drugs to treat diseases of the internal organs—their original self-definition as specialists, before they got turned into a species of generalists. Still others make no distinction at all between the types of primary care providers. Some are quite happy to let your gynecologist attend to all your medical needs. Others are very strict about limiting gynecologists to gynecological problems only.

Your choice of hospitals is limited to those with which the plan has contracted. Since managed care plans are looking to control costs, these hospitals may not be perceived to be the best ones in the city. Managed care plan administrators learn which hospitals are the least expensive and have the best records for particular diseases and types of patients. You may find that you are admitted to one hospital for treatment of one condition and then transferred to another hospital for treatment of a second. If you need specialized surgery, you may have the surgery in a university medical school hospital and be transferred to a small community hospital to recuperate. Saving money in this way enables HMOs to offer the "Cadillac plan" at a rate that employers, patients—and Medicare—are willing to pay.

The opposite side of the coin, of course, is the risk that doctors who contract with managed care plans may be tempted to undertreat people to save money. There have been instances in which managed care plans prevented doctors from telling plan members about highly effective treatments because the cost of such treatments was more than the managed care plan was willing to spend. Fortunately, measures have been taken to correct the situation. Witness the many states that have passed managed care legislation aimed at protecting members. The federal government has also recognized this as a potential problem for beneficiaries and has taken appropriate action. Medicare regulations now prohibit managed care plans from imposing what are called "gag clauses"—clauses in which the plans prohibit their contracted physicians from sharing all relevant health care information with their patients. With the elimination of gag clauses, doctors are obligated to tell you exactly the type of care you need.

In general, studies of patients enrolled in managed care plans have found that their health is just as good as, and perhaps a little bit better than, the health of patients treated by doctors in private practice. Studies have also shown that the quality of care provided by managed care doctors is, in the main, just as good as, or just a little bit better than, the care given by doctors in private practice.

A major disadvantage of managed care plans, for those who travel a good deal, is their reluctance to cover health care other than severe emergencies outside of their service area. If your managed care plan is in North Dakota and you are vacationing in Florida, you can expect that it will cover an emergency room visit for something serious, but not a trip to a local doctor for a cold. Many managed care plans provide a toll-free number to call for preapproval of treatment.

HCFA is listening to the complaints of beneficiaries and is now experimenting with out-of-area coverage. The national Blue Cross and Blue Shield Association has arranged for temporary membership at its member managed care plans for Medicare managed care beneficiaries who live in different parts of the country for a period of time. Unfortunately, this option is not yet available everywhere. Check with the managed care plans you are considering to determine whether they offer this option.

If your managed care plan doesn't offer out-of-area coverage and you still want to travel, you should take note of the many "storefront" medical treatment offices that have opened around the country. While traveling you may wish to use these emergency care centers for treatment of nonsevere illnesses.

Coverage in a Managed Care Plan

The big advantage of managed care plans, given our assumptions about what you want, is that all but a trivial portion of care is prepaid. There are no worries about having the cash to go into the hospital. There are no service-specific charges, so there is no need to negotiate with the doctor about taking assignment. There are far fewer—if any—forms to fill out. One payment covers everything.

Managed care plans usually offer high-option and low-option plans. A typical high-option plan may include all physician services for any purpose; all drugs for any purpose with no, or a small, copayment; unlimited hospital care; all emergency care and all outpatient care; and pediatric services, eyeglasses and hearing aids. Low-option plans vary widely. An increasingly common one entails small copayment—$5 to $10—for everything. This greatly simplifies the managed care plan's bookkeeping and billing operations. It can mean, however, that you owe $200 to $300 for a big day that included a visit with the primary care physician, a referral to a specialist, lab tests, a special x-ray series, a visit to the managed care nurse for shots and treatment and five or six prescriptions. Even so, this is a very small amount compared with the out-of-pocket expenses for a Medicare beneficiary with no supplemental insurance or a plan that imposes heavy copayments and deductibles.

In some managed care plans, the low option is limited to only the services covered by Medicare, but with the managed care plan covering all of Medicare copayments and deductibles and imposing none of its own.

Premiums vary greatly depending on the package of services chosen; the managed care plan's experience with Medicare patients; the number of Medicare beneficiaries versus the number of younger (and usually healthier) people, who are less expensive to care for, enrolled; the hospitals the managed care plan contracts with; going rates for doctors in the area; and so on. Managed care enrollment is growing rapidly, and managed care plans are experimenting with ways to enroll and retain people. Clearly, shopping around, especially where there are competing plans, can be to your advantage. It is safe to say that you will always be able to obtain all the care you need from managed care providers less expensively than with a supplemental insurance plan and certainly less expensively than the cost of Medicare Part B premiums plus the copayments and deductibles.

You continue to pay the Part B premium, and you may also have to pay a premium for services that Medicare does not cover. This extra premium may be larger or smaller than the Part B premium. It is just like the premium you pay for supplemental medical insurance.

Depending on the costs of medical care in your area and the particular managed care plan and options you pick, the individual managed care plan premium may range from a few dollars to around $100 per month. You've probably seen newspaper ads or billboards touting the merits of a Medicare managed care plan with "zero" premiums and added benefits, too!

Conditions for Enrollment as a Medicare Beneficiary

In order to enroll in a managed care plan as a Medicare beneficiary:

- You must be enrolled in both Part A and Part B of Medicare.

- You can join only a managed care plan that has a contract with Medicare.

- You must continue to pay your Medicare Part B monthly premium.

- You must live in the service area of the managed care plan—that is, the geographical area from which the managed care plan is licensed to enroll members.

- You must enroll during your annual coordinated election period or when you first become eligible for Medicare.

- You may withdraw from a managed care plan at any time through the year 2001 by notifying the plan in writing on a form it provides for this purpose. You must submit the withdrawal request by the 10th day of the month in order to return to regular Medicare or a different Medicare+Choice plan on the first of the next month. Requests received after the 10th result in a return to the regular program or a different Medicare+Choice plan on the first of the month after next. In either case, the managed care plan continues to provide you with services until you select another Medicare+Choice plan. Beginning in 2002, you may change plans only once during the first six months of the year. In 2003, this period is reduced to the first three months of the year.

- You cannot be denied enrollment because of your state of health unless you are currently receiving renal dialysis or hospice care. The managed care plan is allowed to deny high-option coverage to persons with some medical conditions.

- All Medicare-covered services must be available with reasonable promptness when needed. Emergency facilities must be available around the clock.

- The managed care plan cannot terminate your membership because of poor health or because of the cost of treating you.

- If the managed care plan ends its contract with Medicare—thereby dropping all Medicare beneficiaries—you must be given at least 60 days' notice. Once you receive this notice, you may join another managed care plan or select another Medicare+Choice option. You must also be given the option of purchasing supplemental insurance without any waiting period for preexisting conditions.

- The managed care plan must have written procedures for resolving complaints.

- You have the right to a 14-day review cycle when you appeal a treatment decision made by your managed care plan. You also have the right to an expedited 72-hour appeal in urgent or emergency situations.

The Big Picture

The premium for a managed care plan that offers additional medical services may seem high, but remember: You are likely to spend 15 percent or more of your income on medical care and supplemental insurance. The managed care plan, in contrast to traditional Medigap insurance, picks up many out-of-pocket expenses that you would otherwise have to pay. More important is the peace of mind you have in knowing that the premium is the only cost, except for nominal copayments. The proper comparison of two insurance plans is always this: *Compare premiums plus out-of-pocket costs for one plan with premiums plus out-of-pocket costs for the other.*

You need to take your time when comparing coverage from various managed care plans. Therefore, we suggest that you make several copies of the worksheets from pages 67-69. Complete the information requested based on what the plan representative told you or the material you received concerning the plan. Whatever you do, *don't* sign up unless all of your questions are answered and you know exactly how the plan works. There's nothing worse than signing up for a managed care plan only to learn that the medical services delivered are far fewer than you expected. But remember: You can withdraw and select another Medicare+Choice plan provided you do so within enrollment periods.

Summing Up Managed Care

Here are some pros and cons to consider before joining a Medicare managed care plan.

The pros:

- All but a small portion of care is prepaid.

- You do not need a supplemental insurance policy.

- More services may be covered than under traditional Medicare coverage.

- Overall out-of-pocket expenses may be lower than the expenses with traditional Medicare coverage and a supplemental policy.

- There are no claims to file; thus, there is less paperwork.

- You can drop out in any given month (until the regulations change in 2002).

- You cannot be denied enrollment because of your state of health (except for the conditions listed earlier).

- Your membership cannot be terminated because of poor health or the cost of treatment.

The cons:

- Your choice of doctors is generally limited to those who contract with the managed care plan (unless you select a POS option).

- Your choice of hospitals is generally limited to those that contract with the managed care plan.

- You may not receive the level of care you want when you want it.

- Some managed care plans won't cover health care (other than emergencies) outside of their service area, and many require out-of-area care to be preapproved. (Some plans offer guest membership arrangements.)

Managed care plans aren't the only options available under the Medicare+Choice program. Congress also directed that Medicare beneficiaries be permitted to experiment with private fee-for-service plans and medical savings accounts.

Of all the new options available to Medicare beneficiaries, private contracting and medical savings accounts are probably the least understood. For this reason, we caution you against making a hasty decision and urge you to carefully weigh the financial advantages and disadvantages of both. Use the worksheet on pages 67-69 to not only evaluate the coverage provided by these plans but also estimate their financial cost.

Private Fee-For-Service Plans (PFFSPs)

PFFSPs pose the most risk for Medicare beneficiaries. Not only do you waive your right to have Medicare pay for your medical services, but you also agree to pay the provider a higher fee than if you were still covered by Medicare. In addition, both you and the physician you privately contract with agree not to submit any claims to Medicare even if the service provided is covered by Medicare.

Under a PFFSP, you contract with physicians and other practitioners for the services you need. Your coverage is provided by an indemnity insurance plan and not Medicare. The insurance plan, not Medicare, sets the reimbursement rate, which may or may not be fully acceptable to the provider. If it isn't, then you pay the difference between what the insurance plan pays and what the provider actually charges.

Furthermore, if you're in a private plan, you may not be able to purchase supplemental insurance to cover any unpaid expenses (see chapter 4). It's also unclear if coverage provided by an employee or retiree health plan covers the difference in reimbursement between the

Medicare-approved payment and the actual charge submitted by the provider. (This issue is currently being decided, and no decision has been reached as this publication goes to press.)

If you select a private plan, Medicare pays the premium for the insurance policy up to an amount equal to the **adjusted average per capita cost (AAPCC)** of providing care to a Medicare beneficiary. For example, if the AAPCC in your area is $500 per month, then Medicare contributes $500 per month toward the purchase of the private plan. If the premium is more than $500 a month, then you make up the difference.

Medicare regulations mandate the following conditions for any private contract:

- The contract must be in writing, and it must be signed by you or your legal representative.

- It must clearly indicate that the physician or practitioner is excluded from participating in the Medicare program (physicians agree not to participate in Medicare for a period of two years).

- It must clearly indicate that neither you nor your legal representative may submit a claim to Medicare even if such service is covered by Medicare. You further agree not to ask a physician or practitioner to submit a claim for you.

- You acknowledge that your **Medigap** insurance or any other supplemental insurance does not or may choose not to make payment for any services you receive (see chapter 4).

- You agree to be responsible for payment of all services received.

- You agree that no reimbursement is provided by Medicare for any services received.

- You agree that the physician or practitioner is not limited in the amount you are charged for services provided.

Signing a private contract for medical services should be done only after you have given the subject serious thought. You might want to discuss this option with an insurance counselor at your local Area Agency on Aging (check the "Guide to Social Services" section of your telephone directory for the listing).

Medical Savings Accounts (MSAs)

MSAs are an experiment that begins this year and runs though the year 2002. Congress has limited the number of MSAs to 390,000, or about 1 percent of the Medicare population.

An MSA is essentially a high deductible, catastrophic insurance policy with a savings account. When you choose a Medicare MSA plan, Medicare pays the premium up to a certain dollar amount and deposits any excess funds into your medical savings account. You have the right to deposit up to $6,000 of your own funds in the MSA.

The amount Medicare is willing to pay is based on the adjusted average per capita cost for a beneficiary. If the average amount is $6,000 and your insurance policy costs $3,000, Medicare pays the premium and deposits $3,000 in your MSA.

You then use the money in your MSA to pay for your medical care until you reach the deductible, at which time the catastrophic insurance plan pays for your care. Unlike original Medicare or one of the managed care options, there are no limits on what providers can charge above the amount paid by the Medicare MSA plan. If at the end of the year there's still money in your MSA, you may withdraw it or let it accumulate tax free from year to year.

Unless you are very wealthy and need to shelter income from taxes, a Medicare MSA plan is probably not for you. Since this is a new program and there's still some question as to the types of insurance plans that will be on the market, be very careful when considering this option.

Selecting a Medicare+Choice Plan

We suggest that at a minimum you acquaint yourself with exactly what is covered by Medicare Parts A and B. A good way to do this is to study the chart on pages 46-47. Also, study the worksheets on pages 67-69 so you are familiar with what you're asked to complete. These worksheets will help you evaluate the coverage offered by original Medicare or any of the Medicare+Choice plans.

Contact the plans in your area and request the schedule of benefits that describes in detail the services covered. Each plan must offer uniform **benefits and premiums** and cost-sharing to all Medicare beneficiaries throughout its service area. Use the worksheets that follow and list each plan and the coverage it provides. Pay particular attention to the extent of coverage in terms of meeting the standards of basic

Medicare coverage (hospital, doctor and laboratory), which they are required to do, and any services that Medicare doesn't cover.

List the monthly premium for the plan, if there is one, or the copayment for the office visit or service provided. Sometimes you are responsible for a copayment of $15 for an office visit or $35 for an emergency department visit. Look for this type of information in the schedule of benefits that comes with the plan. On an exceptionally busy day, as we mentioned, you could encounter several different copayments. Keep a running tally of these out-of-pocket expenses so you know just how much you are spending.

Check the list of providers. Is your primary care doctor part of the plan? Are any of your specialists part of the plan? Is your preferred hospital part of the plan? Are your preferred laboratories and ambulatory facilities part of the plan? These are very important items when considering the quality of care provided and your access to services.

Ask about the internal and external appeals and grievance procedures. Medicare+Choice plans are required to tell you about the time frames for appeals and your rights to have the peer review organization intervene. And finally, ask about the number of doctors who are board certified and how many years they have been in practice. Remember: it's your health at stake and you have every right to ask these important questions.

Use the blank space on the worksheet to record additional questions or make notes on particular plans.

After you have collected all the pertinent information, *take your time in making your decision.* While you may still change your plan coverage from month to month (until the new election and enrollment periods go into effect), this is no way to ensure that you're getting the best quality health care. If in doubt, ask more questions or consult with an insurance counselor at your local senior center or contact the local Area Agency on Aging for assistance.

MEDICARE+CHOICE PLAN WORKSHEET

Use the information provided by the plan to complete this worksheet.

Company Name	Plan 1	Plan 2	Plan 3
Plan Name			
Premium: May be affected by age and sex			
Monthly	$	$	$
Quarterly	$	$	$
Semiannually	$	$	$
Annually	$	$	$
Does the plan cover the deductibles and copayments listed below?	If so, place a checkmark in the appropriate column for each plan.		
Medicare Part A: Hospital			
Initial deductible* $			
61st to 90th Day Copayment* $ /day			
91st to 150th Day Copayment* $ /day			
100% of Medicare-approved expenses for additional 365 days			
Skilled Nursing Care 21st to 100th Day Copayment* $ /day			
Medicare Part B: Physician			
Initial deductible $100			
20% Copayment			
Does the plan provide coverage for the following services?	If so, place a checkmark in the appropriate column for each plan.		
Prescription drugs			
Private duty nursing			
Additional physicians' fees			
Skilled Nursing Care			
Number of days available	_____	_____	_____
Preventive services			
Emergency services (travel)			

*Fill in amounts from current benefit year.

MEDICARE+CHOICE PLAN WORKSHEET, CONT'D

Section I: Organization/Facilities	Plan 1	Plan 2	Plan 3
Travel time to primary care site			
Advance time to make appointments			
Telephone access to primary care doctor			
Emergency care procedure			
Out-of-area care procedure			
Cleanliness of facility			
Modern in appearance			
Staff behavior toward patients			
Patient waiting time			
Health promotion classes (list the type available if any)			
Member grievance process			
Years in business			
Federally qualified			
Other factors: _____ _____ _____			
Section II: Primary Care Physician			
Physician's name			
Specialty board certified			
Years in practice/Years in plan			
Partners/Backup coverage			
Use of physicians' assistants, nurse practitioners, etc.			
Prevention oriented			
Average time spent with patients			
Prescribes generic drugs			
Uses extraordinary life-saving measures			
Admits to hospital			
Communicates well with patients			
Other:_____			

MEDICARE+CHOICE PLAN WORKSHEET, CONT'D

Section III: Backup System	Plan 1	Plan 2	Plan 3
Additional hospitals in plan			
Travel time to each			
Second opinion surgical program			
Referrals to non-plan specialists			
Quality assurance program			
Procedure for changing primary care doctor			

Additional notes:

In this chapter you will learn: When you are not responsible for the cost of services received ■ When you are responsible for the cost of services received ■ What is meant by deductibles and copayments ■ How to read a Medicare Summary Notice ■ What is covered by Medicare Part A (hospital insurance) ■ What is meant by benefit period ■ How the Diagnosis-Related Groups system affects hospital payments and you ■ What your rights are while a hospital patient ■ What is covered by Medicare Part B (doctor insurance)

3. What Medicare Does (and Doesn't) Pay For

The purpose of this chapter is to explain, in terms that are as clear as the complexity of the program permits, exactly what Medicare pays for and what you (or your insurer or both) have to pay for.

Medicare makes either full or partial payments for a wide range of health care services. When a partial payment is made, it means you are usually responsible for a deductible and copayment. Even if you have insurance that supplements Medicare, the insurance plan may require you to pay part of the cost. The same may be true if you belong to one of the Medicare+Choice plans, especially if you've selected a private fee-for-service plan (PFFSP) or medical savings account (MSA) plan. The phrase "what you pay for" in this chapter should be understood to include what has to be paid, regardless of who pays it. You may have other sources of payment for what Medicare doesn't cover—payments made by your insurer or Medicare+Choice plan (plus what you pay out of pocket).

What gets paid for, how much and when, under Medicare, is an odd combination of the following:

- The *services* that providers agree to provide in their contracts with Medicare

- The *amount* of the services that Medicare covers

- Medicare's commitment to *cost-sharing* through a deductible (an amount you must pay before coverage begins) and a copayment (an amount you pay when you receive a service)

- How *the law* establishing Medicare (Title XVIII of the Social Security Act) dictates that each type of provider be paid

- The *medical necessity* of the services you actually received

Unfortunately, the regulations that govern Medicare do not break down what is paid for, how much and when into these terms. As a result, it is very difficult to discover exactly what is paid or not paid and under what conditions by reading them. But the ways we have cut them up, above, really do cover all the issues that are involved in determining what you wind up paying for. In the appropriate sections, which begin on page 77, we discuss what Medicare pays and what you pay under the following related headings:

- Limitations on Services

- Cost-Sharing

- How Payment Is Made

- Medical Necessity Determinations

When You Never Have to Pay

There are numerous situations in which Medicare decides not to pay a provider or to pay less than the provider wanted. It's important to understand when you don't have to pay for something that Medicare has refused to pay a provider for. *You are never obligated to pay for a service unless you can reasonably have been expected to know that the service was not covered or was not medically reasonable and necessary. You are never obligated to pay more than Medicare has decided to pay the provider if the provider has agreed to accept assignment.*

"Reasonably Have Been Expected to Know"

"Reasonably have been expected to know" is a legal phrase. What it means, basically, is this: If you have not been *informed in writing* by an appropriate review authority (the provider, a Medicare intermediary or carrier or Medicare itself) that a service is not covered or is not medically reasonable and necessary and you could not be expected to know it from official sources (such as pamphlets that you were given when you signed up for Medicare or prior notices that such services were not covered), then you do not have to pay for it, even if Medicare doesn't. The key word is "reasonably." What you can reasonably be expected to know is that which a reasonable person would expect an individual like you, in your situation, having received the information you received, to know. The working definition, as Medicare's administrative law judges and the courts use it, resides in case law and is continuously evolving. As stated in the regulations, there are two important parts: You have to receive a written notice, and you have to receive it from *an appropriate source.*

Some examples may help here:

Example 1: *You go into the hospital for surgery. The operation (or procedure; we'll call all procedures "operations" for the sake of simplicity) is one that Medicare normally requires be done in an outpatient facility (a clinic, an **ambulatory surgery** center or the doctor's office) because it has been proven that this can be done safely and at lower cost than in the hospital. Your doctor believes that he can show that your case requires inpatient surgery. The peer review organization (PRO) that reviews such cases disagrees. The hospital gets paid nothing by Medicare, but you do not have to pay anything either. Why? Because you cannot reasonably have been expected to know exactly which operations are required to be done as outpatient operations or the steps your doctor should have followed to check.*

Example 2: *You go into the hospital for surgery. The operation is one that Medicare normally requires be done only after a PRO has approved it. (This may be because there is disagreement among doctors about when the operation is needed or whether it works or because there is wide variation across the country in the number of operations done on similar groups of people. It may also be because the PRO has determined that many of the operations performed in your area turn out to be unnecessary.) The hospital does not obtain approval. The hospital is paid nothing by Medicare, but you are not required to pay anything either. Why? You cannot reasonably have been expected to know which operations were on the preapproval list.*

Example 3: *You have carefully searched for a doctor who accepts assignment. The doctor you chose is on the list of **Medicare-participating physicians** that your local Social Security office provided you. You specifically ask her if she takes assignment. She says that she does. The old year passes, and the new one begins. You suddenly begin getting bills from her for more than 20 percent of Medicare's charge for her services.*

*It turns out that she has not renewed her **participating physician agreement** with Medicare and has taken no steps to inform her patients. You call the office to complain and find out that she no longer accepts assignment. You do not have to pay more than 20 percent of the **Medicare-approved charge** until you learn this; however, you are required to pay the extra costs for services received after you learn this.*

Example 4: *You are discharged from the hospital but need further therapy before you can go home. You are admitted to a nursing home for some physical therapy and daily changing of a dressing. The PRO determines that you could have been treated at home or at the doctor's office, so your stay is not medically necessary. The nursing home is paid nothing by Medicare, but you do not have to pay anything either. Why? Because you could not have reasonably been expected to know the criteria used to evaluate your case.*

Don't worry if you didn't understand everything in the examples. What you need to understand is the general principle: When Medicare makes a payment, all sorts of wheels turn, about which you cannot reasonably be expected to know. You are protected from the consequences of behind-the-scenes decisions if you are not informed of them. *The fact that Medicare has refused payment doesn't mean that you have to pay.*

On the other hand, there are situations in which you can "reasonably be expected to know" something or other, and you must act to make sure that you do not have to pay more than is necessary. Some examples, parallel to the ones above, should help make this clear:

Example 1: *You go into the hospital for surgery. The operation is one that Medicare normally requires be done in an outpatient facility because it has been proven that this can be done safely and at lower cost than in the hospital. Your doctor believes that he can show that your case requires inpatient surgery. He checks with the appropriate personnel at the hospital. They advise him that your condition does not require hospitalization and can safely be done in an outpatient facility (a clinic, an ambulatory surgery center or the doctor's office). You are informed of this, in writing. However, you do not appeal and instead decide to go to the hospital. As expected, the PRO recommends that nothing be paid for the hospital stay. You are so informed, in writing. You do not appeal. You have to pay the hospital bill and any doctor bills associated with having the operation in the hospital. Why? You could reasonably have been expected to know that this operation was required to be done as an outpatient operation; you were informed in writing.*

Example 2: You go into the hospital for surgery. The operation is one that Medicare normally requires be done only after the PRO has approved it. The hospital does not obtain approval. Your doctor tells you this, in writing. *You do not insist that a formal determination be made, or one is made and you do not appeal it. You decide to go ahead with the operation. You have to pay the hospital bill plus any additional doctor fees. Why? You could reasonably have been expected to know that Medicare would not pay for the operation; you were informed in writing.*

Example 3: You have carefully searched for a doctor who accepts assignment. The doctor you chose is on the list of Medicare-participating physicians that your local Social Security office provided you. You specifically ask her if she takes assignment. She says that she does. The old year passes, and the new one begins. The doctor informs all her patients, in writing, *by letter, that she will no longer accept assignment for all Medicare patients. You suddenly begin getting bills from her for more than the 20 percent of the Medicare-approved charge. Are you responsible for the additional amount over and above the 20 percent copayment? Yes. Why? Because you could have reasonably been expected to know that the physician no longer accepts assignment since you were informed in writing. However, you are protected from excessive* **balance billing** *by a Medicare regulation that limits what the physician may charge you.*

Medicare regulations limit the maximum fee that a nonparticipating physician may charge you and the amount of balance billing that he may do. Using the Medicare-approved amount as the base, a physician's maximum fee for a service is limited to a markup of 115 percent. You do not have to pay any amount that exceeds the maximum charge.

Example 4: You are discharged from the hospital but need further therapy before you can go home. You are admitted to a nursing home for some physical therapy and daily changing of a dressing. The PRO determines that you could have been treated at home or at the doctor's office, so your stay is not considered medically necessary. You are informed of this, in writing, *and you elect not to appeal the decision or you lose your appeal. You have to pay for the nursing home stay. Why? You could reasonably have been expected to know that Medicare would not pay; you were informed in writing.*

Again, don't worry about the technicalities here. We inform you about what you can appeal, and how to do it, later. Chapter 8 provides more detail about the appeal process. For the moment, remember three things:

- First, an oral notice to you isn't worth anything. Only written notifications have effect.

- Second, the written notice must come from an appropriate source: the PRO, the Medicare intermediary or carrier or the provider (doctor, hospital or nursing home official).

- Third, once you have been informed that a service is not covered, you are expected to know that it is not covered in the future.

Dealing With Claims, Bills and Carriers

We aren't saying that hospitals and doctors are unethical, but—like most of us—they prefer getting money to not getting money. They do not see it as their job to determine exactly what has and hasn't been approved and bill you only for your share of the approved charges. However, a recent change in Medicare regulations does make doctors— even those who do not accept Medicare assignment—responsible for filing all Medicare claims. However, we recommend that you use the **Medicare Summary Notice (MSN)**—see sample on pages 78-79—sent to you by the Medicare carrier and the information you receive from your insurance company to keep track of claims in the event of a problem.

The intermediaries and carriers who handle Medicare payments see it as their primary duty to get the checks and the bills out. The PRO is interested in making determinations of medical necessity and arguing with Medicare to get more money in its next review contract. *So none of these parties has as its main concern making sure that you get billed for only what you really have to pay. You have to look out for yourself.* Because the payment system under Medicare is so complicated, it is virtually certain that at least one of your encounters with a health care provider will result in a bill for something you don't really owe. Because of this same complexity, and because there can be a considerable time lag before your case is reviewed (if it needs to be) or the hospital is audited, a long time can pass before who has to pay for what is finally decided.

Your Medicare carrier or intermediary is required, as part of its contract with Medicare, to maintain a mailing address to which you can write about amounts you think you don't owe. Most of them also provide a telephone number. Your Medicare supplemental insurance carrier should have such an address and a telephone number and is usually required by state insurance laws to have both. (Telephone numbers of the various Medicare intermediaries and carriers are provided in appendix A.) Your managed care plan, if you belong to one, is required by both state and federal laws to have a procedure for resolving disputes. If your dispute cannot be settled within the plan, you may request assistance from the **Center for Health Dispute Resolution (CHDR)**. Your plan must provide you with the information on how to contact the CHDR (pronounced "cheddar"). If it doesn't, telephone the Medicare information line at 800-638-6833.

Services Covered Under Part A of Medicare

Hospitals

You may want to examine the Medicare coverage chart on pages 46-47 before reading any further. We want to call your attention to the column labeled "benefit period."

A benefit period is a way of measuring your use of services under Medicare hospital insurance. Your first benefit period starts when you enter a hospital and after your hospital coverage begins. A benefit period ends when you have been out of the hospital or other facility (skilled nursing facility or rehabilitation center) for 60 days.

It's very important that you understand the benefit period because it will help you determine when you are liable for the one-day Part A deductible. For example, if you are admitted to the hospital for the first time on January 15 and are discharged on January 25, you would pay the Part A deductible. If you are readmitted on February 5, you do not pay the deductible because it has been less than 60 days since your previous hospitalization, and your readmission date is day 11 in your benefit period.

On the other hand, if you are not hospitalized again until October 1 and are discharged on October 23, you are liable for the one-day Part A deductible because more than 60 days have elapsed since your previous hospitalization.

Medicare's discussion of covered services for hospitals is basically an attempt to describe, at length, the services that hospitals normally provide to all patients. Bed and board, nursing services, use of hospital facilities, medical social services, drugs, biologicals, use of supplies and equipment, diagnostic and therapeutic services and the services of house staff (interns and residents in training) are covered.

Limitations on Services: Private rooms are not covered unless your medical condition requires you to be isolated or unless there are no semiprivate or ward rooms available. Medicare pays until you no longer

HCFA

Medicare Summary Notice

June 16, 1996 ①

CUSTOMER SERVICE INFORMATION ②

BENEFICIARY NAME ④
STREET ADDRESS
CITY, STATE ZIP CODE

③ ➤ **Your Medicare Number: 111-11-1111A**

If you have questions, write or call:
Medicare
555 Medicare Blvd.
Suite 200
Medicare Building
Medicare, US XXXXX-XXXX

Local: (XXX) XXX-XXXX
Toll-free: 1-800-XXX-XXXX
Tele-Device for the Deaf: 1-800-XXX-XXXX

⑤ **HELP STOP FRAUD**: Protect your Medicare Number as you would a credit card number.

This is a summary of claims processed from 5/15/96 through 6/15/96.

⑥ PART A HOSPITAL INSURANCE - INPATIENT CLAIMS

Dates of Service ⑦	Benefit Days Used ⑧	Amount Charged ⑨	Non-Covered Charges ⑩	Deductible and Coinsurance ⑪	You May Be Billed ⑫	See Notes Section ⑬
Care Hospital, 124 Sick Lane **Dallas, TX 75555** ⑭						
Referred by: Paul Jones, M.D.						
04/25/96-05/09/96	14 days	$14,732.23	$0.00	$736.00	$736.00	a.b

① The **Date** the MSN was sent.

② Refer to the **Customer Service Information** box if you have questions about your MSN. For all inquiries, include your Medicare number, the date of the notice, and the specific date of service you have questions about.

③ **Your Medicare Number** should match the number on your Medicare card.

④ If your **Name and Address** are incorrect on your MSN, please contact the Medicare intermediary shown on your MSN immediately.

⑤ Read the **Help Stop Fraud** message for information on ways to protect yourself and Medicare against fraud and abuse.

⑥ **Part A Hospital Insurance - Inpatient Claims** or **Part B Medical Insurance - Outpatient Claims**. The Inpatient claims (for hospitals and skilled nursing facilities) and Outpatient claims are listed separately.

⑦ **Dates of Service** shows when services were provided.

⑧ **Benefit Days Used** shows the number of days used in the benefit period. See the back of your MSN for an explanation of benefit period.

Note: For Part B Medical Insurance - Outpatient Facility Claims (not shown here), the column will be titled **Services Provided** and will give a brief description of the service or supply provided.

⑨ **Amount Charged** is the charge submitted to Medicare by the provider of service(s).

⑩ **Non-Covered Charges** shows the charges for services denied or excluded by the Medicare program for which you may be billed.

⑪ The amount applied to your **Deductible and Coinsurance**.

⑫ **You May Be Billed.** This is the total amount the provider is allowed to bill you. It combines the deductible, the coinsurance and any non-covered charges. If you have supplemental insurance, it may pay all or part of this amount.

⑬ **See Notes Section.** If a letter appears in this column, refer to the Notes Section. Please see item 15 in this pamphlet.

⑭ **Provider's Name and Address** shows the name of the facility where you received services. The referring doctor's name will also be shown. The address shown is the billing address which may be different from where you received the service(s).

(15) **Notes Section:**

a You have 46 full days remaining in this benefit period.

b $736.00 was applied to your inpatient deductible.

(16) **Deductible Information:**

You have met the Part A deductible for this benefit period.

(17) **General Information:**

Please notify us if your address has changed or is incorrect as shown on this notice.

Appeals Information - Part A (Inpatient)   (18)

If you disagree with any claims decision on PART A of this notice, you can request an appeal by August 16, 1996. Follow the instructions below:

- Circle the item(s) you disagree with and explain why you disagree.
- Send this notice, or a copy, to the address in the "Customer Service Information" box on Page 1.
- Sign here _____ Phone number (___) _____

Appeals Information - Part B (Outpatient)

If you disagree with any claims decision on PART B of this notice, you can request an appeal by December 16, 1996. Follow the instructions below:

(18) **Appeals Information**, such as how and when to request an appeal, is shown here. See the back of your MSN for more information and how to get help with appeal requests.

Note: The Medicare Handbook provides more information about coverage and other services. For a free copy, call the Medicare contractor listed in the Customer Service box on your MSN.

☆ U.S. GOVERNMENT PRINTING OFFICE 1996 706 415

(15) The **Notes Section** gives more detailed information about your claim.

(16) The **Deductible Information** section shows how much of your Part A and/or Part B deductible has been met.

(17) The **General Information** section provides important Medicare news and information.

need the private room or until you can be transferred to a semiprivate room or ward. You do not have to pay for the private room unless it was requested by you or a member of your family who was told, at the time the request was made, that there would be an additional charge. (Please note that the notice here does not need to be a written one.)

Medicare does not pay for the services of a private duty nurse unless the hospital normally provides one for patients in your condition.

Medicare pays for drugs used only while in the hospital. However, the hospital may give you a limited supply of drugs to take with you if this will facilitate your discharge and the drug is needed until you can obtain a continuing supply.

Medicare pays for all supplies and equipment used in the hospital. It pays for supplies taken out of the hospital for outpatient use only if use must continue after you leave (such as a pacemaker) or the supplies are required to assist your departure (such as crutches).

The chart on pages 46-47 should make it obvious that there is a good reason to have some Medicare supplemental insurance, especially if you've elected to remain in the original Medicare program. Beneficiaries who select one of the managed care options may not need to worry about carrying supplemental insurance. We discuss how to find and evaluate supplemental insurance in chapter 4.

Cost-Sharing: When you are admitted to the hospital, Medicare requires that you pay a one-day deductible of several hundred dollars. If your hospital stay lasts at least 61 days, you are also responsible for daily copayments, which continue until you are discharged.

How Payment Is Made: Payment for hospitals under Medicare has always been complicated. It has recently gotten more so because of changes to the Medicare law passed by Congress that established the **prospective payment** system for hospitals. Prospective payments to hospitals are made through the Diagnosis-Related Groups (DRG) system.

Why Prospective Payment? Consider an example. Suppose you go to an auto dealer and ask whether you need a car. If the answer is yes, you want the dealer to decide what kind of car a person like you should have, get it for you and bill you, without regard to price. The chances are you will get a Mercedes, with all the options. Consider another example. You go to the car dealer and say, "I want a compact car with all-weather radial tires, a stereo cassette deck and air-conditioning. I want it in black. It has to have at least a 50,000-mile guarantee on all major parts and the body. I know cars like this can be bought for no more than $12,500. Get me the car, and I will pay you that, but no more." Chances are that you will get what you want, for no more than $12,500. The dealer will try to get a higher price, and you will have to negotiate, but you will get the car you specified.

Any insurer—including Medicare—that makes **retrospective payments** to a health care provider is in the first situation. (Retrospective payments are made after a service has been rendered. Retrospective payment is the traditional system of payment in the United States, although this is changing.) In this **fee-for-service system**, in which providers render whatever services they think are necessary and then bill for them, there is a danger of getting much more than is needed and paying more than is really necessary. You are also in danger of being told that you need a car when you really don't. In the second situation, you are protected: You have made the decision that you want the car, and you will not buy it at more than the agreed-upon price. This is the benefit of prospective payment, especially with appropriate controls such as second opinions on surgery and the requirement of preapproval for some operations and hospital stays. Providers argue constantly about the evils of prospective payment, but there is considerable research evidence that shows that the quality of care need not suffer and that providers can make a good profit under it.

Congress required that Medicare pay for hospital services under Medicare via a prospective payment scheme because it was convinced that this step would help avoid unnecessary hospitalization and control costs. Prospective payment protects you.

The Diagnosis-Related Groups System

The DRG system is Medicare's current method of prospective payment. It was developed originally by the Yale School of Organization and Management and became law for hospitals in the state of New Jersey before Congress made it national law for Medicare. Using sophisticated statistical techniques, Medicare cases were analyzed to see how payments should be set to cover as many cases as possible. This research showed that the main or **primary diagnosis** of the patient, **secondary diagnoses**, age and performed operations predicted costs for the majority of patients quite well. The billions of possible combinations of these factors were reduced to 495 DRGs, each of which is best understood as an overall condition of a patient. Congress understood that these 495 groups would not cover every case, and they made provisions for **outliers**—people who needed more days in the hospital or more expensive hospital stays because they had illnesses or needed operations that resulted in a stay that exceeded the length assigned by the DRG system. Hospitals can be granted payment for cases that require more hospital days than predicted by the DRG system, provided the continued stay is medically necessary. Cases that do not exceed the length of stay criteria but are more costly than predicted by a certain amount are paid more if the hospital applies for additional payment.

The Diagnosis-Related Groups System, Hospitals and You: The DRG system was phased in over several years, and today virtually every general, acute care hospital in the country is paid with the DRG system.

The way it works is as follows: You are admitted to the hospital as a Medicare patient. Your DRG cannot be assigned when you come in because your diagnosis may be unknown or wrong. Also, the operations that you will have cannot be predicted in advance, especially if you are admitted only for a **diagnostic workup**. Once everything has been done and you are ready to be discharged, the hospital prepares a **face sheet** for your hospital chart that indicates your DRG. The DRG will probably have been assigned by a computer program that was purchased by the hospital and designed to pick the highest-paid DRG possible, based on your combination of age, diagnoses, operations and other factors. The Medicare intermediary pays the hospital the DRG rate after a computer review of the hospital's DRG coding.

Note that the hospital couldn't assign the DRG when you came in and, therefore, could not predict the cost of your care or how much it would be paid. The result is that on some admissions the hospital loses money and on some admissions it makes money. On the average, hospitals that are generally as "good"—measured by their use of resources on patients, not by the results they produce—as the average hospital break even. Those that are better in this sense make money, and they are allowed to keep their profits. Those that are worse lose money, and they have to swallow their losses.

The important point is this: *There is no guarantee from Medicare that the hospital will not lose or make money on your case. Its loss or gain, under the DRG system, is supposed to have nothing to do with your care.*

Let's look at some examples:

You are over 75 years old, have a minor heart attack, fall down a flight of stairs as a result and break a hip. The surgeon decides that a total hip replacement is needed. You have the operation. Much to everyone's surprise, there are no complications, and you quickly learn to walk with the artificial hip and are able to go home well before the DRG-assigned number of hospital days. The hospital makes money on your case and gets to keep it.

Now imagine the same circumstances, but (as might be expected given this situation) your care is long and difficult, and complications arise. You develop thrombophlebitis in your legs and have to have more surgery and additional drugs. You have a bleeding episode as a result of the drugs and need a transfusion. You are very weak and take a long time to get to the point at which you can be discharged to a skilled nursing facility to learn to walk again. Even with outlier payments, the hospital loses a great deal of money on your case.

In both these situations, the hospital is supposed to give you care that is medically necessary, regardless of the amount it has to spend.

Results to date suggest that *hospital profits are at their highest level in history,* based largely on profits from Medicare patients. Some types of hospitals such as rural hospitals, inner-city hospitals with large charity care burdens and hospitals that are the sole hospital for large areas seem to be losing money. Congress has required Medicare to watch hospital profits carefully and to report to it, through the Prospective Payment Assessment Commission, on any adjustments that should be made. For the most part, though, the DRG system has been a financial boon to hospitals. Most recent studies show hospital profit margins to be quite healthy, even with the impact of managed care. Fewer hospitals than ever are losing money on prospective payment.

Another point that needs to be understood is this: Since DRG payments are based on national/regional averages, it is *planned* that some hospitals will make money and some will lose money. It's part of the concept. One of the objectives of the DRG system, in fact, was the closure of the nation's least-efficient hospitals. It was hoped that they would lose so much money that they would have to close. Patients would then go to the more-efficient hospitals, and overall costs would be reduced. This is another reason that losses (or profits) made by the hospital under the DRG system should have nothing to do with your care. *These losses (or profits) are a result of the overall efficiency of the hospital, not your particular medical needs. No one case is going to break (or make) a hospital.*

During the early days of the DRG system, there were a number of instances of abuse. Patients were told that they had to leave the hospital because their "DRG has run out" or some similar phrasing. Discharging any patient who still needs hospital care because of financial considerations is a total violation of the hospital's contract with Medicare. The hospital has agreed to provide services to you as long as they are medically necessary.

Because of the abuses that were observed, the People's Medical Society and the American Association of Retired Persons joined forces to ask Medicare to require hospitals to "Mirandize" Medicare patients just as persons being arrested are told of their constitutional rights. Medicare now requires *all* hospitals to provide Medicare beneficiaries with an *Important Message from Medicare* upon admission for any inpatient hospital care. It appears on pages 152-153.

To sum up: The only reasons that you can be discharged from a hospital under Medicare are *medical* ones.

Medical Necessity Determinations: Medicare does not pay for services that are not medically "reasonable and necessary."

Who makes this determination? The first person who comes to mind, obviously, is your doctor. If your doctor suggests that you are ready to go home, you are likely to comply. If you feel you need more time, discuss it with her. The real issue comes when you want to stay in the hospital and the hospital's **utilization review committee (URC)** wants you to leave or the PRO wants you to leave. In either case, you will receive a written notice that a decision has been made and that you have the right to appeal it. How to appeal it is covered in chapter 8.

If you win the appeal, you stay. If you lose, you may be required to pay for up to one day of hospital stay after the original cutoff date. It's important to understand that there are two tracks here, as described in the information on requesting a review given a few pages back. If you are asking the PRO to review the hospital's decision, you are not responsible for services received before you get the notice of the PRO's decision. If you are asking the PRO to rethink its own decision, the hospital may start billing you beginning with the third calendar day after you received the **Notice of Noncoverage**. If the PRO does not reverse its position and you decide not to stay in the hospital, you may have to pay for the third day. If you decide to stay, you are responsible for the further cost of your care.

Beneficiaries enrolled in Medicare+Choice plans also have the right to appeal decisions made by their plans or hospitals that care is no longer needed. As a member of a managed care plan, you have the right to request an expedited PRO review or an expedited review by your plan's internal appeals process.

If you're in a managed care plan, the most significant factor weighing on your decision to appeal is protection from financial liability should you lose. We've already mentioned that you gain extra time in the hospital by appealing to the PRO, and you also gain protection from financial liability until the PRO issues its decision. However, if you request an expedited review from your managed care plan rather than the PRO, *you are not protected from financial liability during your appeal.* Your plan has 72 hours to conduct the expedited review, but by that time you could be responsible for thousands of dollars in hospital charges.

If your plan is unable to reach a decision, your case is sent to the Center for Health Dispute Resolution (CHDR), an organization that contracts with Medicare to review decisions made by managed care plans. We provide more information on appeals in chapter 8.

Skilled Nursing Facilities

Care in a skilled nursing facility is less intense than that you receive in a hospital but more intense than the custodial care provided in an **intermediate care facility** or **custodial care facility**. Basically, all of the services listed under hospitals are covered under skilled nursing facilities. The exceptions are services that skilled nursing facilities do not normally provide, such as surgery. Medicare permits hospitals with fewer than 100 beds that have empty beds to run a skilled nursing facility within their walls, using beds that have been designated as **swing beds**. Swing beds are used as skilled nursing facility beds when there is a need for skilled nursing facility services and as hospital beds when there is a need for hospital services. In effect, the hospital uses part of its capacity as a skilled-nursing-facility-type nursing home.

Limitations on Services: Many people think that Medicare pays for long-term nursing home care. There are sometimes tragic results from confusion about this. *Medicare does not pay for "custodial" or "personal care" services in nursing homes—only for rehabilitative care. This care is limited to 100 days per benefit period.*

Cost-Sharing: You are entitled to 100 days of skilled nursing facility care during each benefit period. Medicare pays all costs for the first 20 days, and beginning on the 21st day, you are responsible for the co-payment of $96 per day. You would pay this until the 100th day, after which you are responsible for all costs. See the following example.

> *After a long and complicated hospital stay, Victoria Smith-Jones is sent to a skilled nursing facility. She does not improve as rapidly as everyone had hoped and has to spend 135 days there. The daily charge is $110. For the first 20 days Medicare covers all costs, and she pays nothing. Beginning on the 21st day and for the next 80 days, her copayment is $96 per day for a total of $7,680. Medicare picks up the extra $14 per day during this 80-day period. For the next 35 days Victoria Smith-Jones is responsible for all costs. Her total charge for the stay in the nursing home is $14,850. Medicare contributed $3,320 toward the total cost.*

How Payment Is Made: The skilled nursing facility (or the hospital that provides skilled nursing facility care in a swing bed) is paid a daily amount by the intermediary, less your coinsurance.

Medical Necessity Determinations: Medical necessity is the *key* issue in payment for skilled nursing facility services. The skilled nursing facility regulations go to great lengths to define what is and is not skilled nursing facility care. The key is that care complex enough to require the services of a nurse or skilled rehabilitation personnel is covered; care that you could handle by yourself is not. But complications may require skilled-nursing-facility-level care, even for situations that would normally not be covered. Basically, skilled nursing facility care is rehabilitation; if your condition cannot be expected to improve as a result of skilled nursing facility care *and* you do not need observation by skilled personnel, your care is not covered. Obviously, what your doctor writes in the chart makes a big difference in what gets covered. If you are worried about coverage of skilled nursing facility services, discuss this with your doctor.

If you receive a written notice from the skilled nursing facility's or the hospital's URC or from the PRO that your condition no longer requires skilled nursing facility services, you can appeal. If you win the appeal, your care is paid for as long as it is medically necessary. If you lose, you pay for all care after the cutoff date. Chapter 8 explains how to appeal decisions regarding coverage related to medical necessity.

Home Health Services

Medicare covers medical services that are needed to allow you to live at home. The scope of benefits includes part-time or intermittent nursing care; physical, occupational or speech therapy; medical social services; part-time or intermittent services of a home health aide; medical supplies; durable medical equipment; and the services of interns and residents if the **home health agency** is affiliated with a teaching hospital. If you continue to need occupational therapy, that is covered, even after the physical or speech therapy is over.

As with skilled nursing facilities, personal care services are not covered. Housekeeping and transportation are not included. To receive home health services, you must be confined to your home or to an institution that is not a nursing home. Being able to take trips to see the doctor or to go to the hospital does not mean that you are not homebound.

Home health care is covered under both Part A (hospital insurance) and Part B (doctor insurance) of Medicare. For coverage, all the following conditions must exist:

- You are confined to your home.
- You need part-time skilled nursing or physical or speech therapy.
- A doctor prescribes home health care.
- The home health agency is approved by Medicare.

Limitations on Services: Home health care is limited to 21 consecutive visits.

Cost-Sharing: There is no cost-sharing under home health care except for the $100 Part B deductible for services furnished under Part B, and 20 percent of the reasonable charge under Part A for durable medical equipment supplied by home health care. The home health agency charges patients for any services provided by it that are not covered under Medicare. You should ask your doctor and the home health agency if any services not covered under Medicare are provided and what the charges will be. Based on what you hear, you may want to discuss your plan of care with your doctor.

How Payment Is Made: Home health agencies bill the Medicare intermediary directly and bill you for any noncovered services.

Medical Necessity Determinations: Your need for continuing home health care must be reviewed periodically by a physician. You will be notified in writing if a finding is made that home health care is no longer medically necessary, and you have appeal rights, which are discussed in chapter 8.

Hospice Services

Hospice care is care provided to those who are **terminally ill**, either in their homes or in hospice facilities. It is designed to help those who are dying do so with the greatest possible dignity and comfort, while avoiding treatment that will only prolong suffering. While the Medicare hospice benefit primarily provides for care at home, it can help pay for inpatient care. In addition, services not usually covered by Medicare, including homemaking, counseling and certain prescription drugs, are covered.

Limitations on Services: Hospice care is available for a total of 210 days, which consists of two 90-day periods and one 30-day period, provided that a physician or the hospice director certifies that the person is still terminally ill.

Cost-Sharing: You are responsible for a copayment on all prescription medications, as well as a daily copayment when you require inpatient care.

How Payment Is Made: Medicare pays nearly the entire cost of hospice care. You are responsible for a copayment on each prescription medication and a daily copayment when inpatient care is required.

Medical Necessity Determinations: Your doctor and the hospice director must certify that you are terminally ill and attest to your continuing need for care. You have the right to appeal to the PRO if you disagree with any treatment decisions made by your doctor or the hospice director.

Respite Care

Respite care is a part of hospice care. Periodically, the hospice may arrange for inpatient care in either a hospital or skilled nursing home to give temporary relief to the primary caregiver.

Limitations on Services: Inpatient care is limited to no more than five days in a row.

Cost-Sharing: You are responsible for a copayment on all prescription medications, as well as 5 percent of the cost up to the Part A deductible.

How Payment Is Made: Medicare covers the entire cost of respite care except for a copayment covering prescription medications and an inpatient copayment.

Medical Necessity Determinations: As with hospice care, your doctor must certify that you require this type of care. You also have the same appeals rights that you do under hospice care.

Blood Services

There is a separate blood deductible for Parts A and B, although the deductible needs to be met only one time. You are responsible for paying for the first three units of whole blood or packed red cells received in a hospital or skilled nursing facility. You must either pay for the blood or have it replaced. You are considered to have replaced it if an acceptable donor offers to replace it on your behalf, whether the provider or its blood supplier accepts the offer. If you have paid for or replaced blood under Part B, you do not need to pay for or replace that blood again under Part A.

Services Covered Under Part B of Medicare

Doctors' Services

Medicare was designed around the Blue Cross/Blue Shield model, which has one part paying for hospital services and another paying for everything else. "Everything else" is the job of Part B of Medicare.

Among the services covered are: physicians' services, outpatient hospital services, diagnostic tests, outpatient physical therapy, speech pathology services, rural health clinic services and outpatient renal dialysis services. Also covered are services furnished by ambulatory surgical centers, home health agencies and comprehensive outpatient rehabilitation facilities, immunosupressive drugs, medical supplies, durable medical equipment and supplies that are not covered under Medicare Part A.

There's also improved coverage for a number of items.

- Mammograms are covered under the following conditions:
  - A patient is 40 years of age or older and desires an annual mammogram. The Part B deductible is waived;
  - A patient has distinct signs and symptoms for which a mammogram is indicated;
  - A patient has a personal or family history of breast cancer; or
  - A patient is asymptomatic but, on the basis of the patient's history and other factors (the physician considers significant), the physician's judgment is that a mammogram is appropriate.

- Enhanced coverage of Pap smears and pelvic examinations for the early detection of cervical cancer are covered, and the Part B deductible is waived. Pap smears are also covered when ordered by a physician under one of the following conditions:
  - A patient has not had a test during the preceding three years; or
  - A patient is at high risk for cervical cancer and her physician recommends that she have the test performed more frequently than every three years.

- Colorectal cancer screenings for beneficiaries age 50 and older are covered.

- Bone mass measurements are covered for individuals at high risk of osteoporosis.

- Diabetes self-management training services, glucose monitors and test strips for people with type 2 diabetes are covered.

- Immunizations, including flu, pneumonia and hepatitis B shots, are covered.

Limitations on Services: The following is a laundry list of limited services:

- Chiropractors' services are limited to 12 treatments unless more are determined to be medically necessary.

- Optometrists' services are limited to testing and examination needed to fit artificial lenses to treat aphakia (absence of the lens of the eye, whether natural or caused by the removal of a cataract).

- Dentists' services and dental surgeons' services are covered only if they would have been covered if performed by a doctor.

- Podiatrists' services are covered only if they would have been covered if performed by a doctor.

- There is a 50 percent copayment on outpatient psychiatric services.

- Ambulance services are covered if the ambulance equipment and personnel meet Medicare requirements and transportation in any other vehicle could endanger your life.

Other exclusions include:

- Over-the-counter drugs

- Most eyeglasses and eye exams

- Hearing aids and fittings

- Full-time nursing care in the home

- Routine physical exams

Also, services paid for by workers' compensation, automobile or other liability insurance, employer health plans (for retirees or current employees, whichever you happen to be) and other government programs are not covered to the extent that these programs pay for the services you receive. Depending on the circumstances and the service, Medicare may pay the difference between what these programs paid and what you owe, but Medicare pays nothing unless you are obligated to make a payment.

Cost-Sharing: Part B is modeled on basic Blue Cross/Blue Shield plans as they existed in the mid-1960s. You are responsible for a $100 annual deductible and 20 percent of the "reasonable cost" of all services. Your 20 percent copayment is based upon the Medicare-approved amount and may not reflect the actual charge for services provided by nonparticipating physicians. There is no cap on your out-of-pocket expenses under Medicare Part B.

How Payment Is Made: Now the fun begins. At one time, Medicare employed the **usual, customary and reasonable** process for determining doctors' payments. One of the things that doctors insisted on in the formulation of the original Blue Shield plans was that they get paid, in essence, what they wanted. This approach worked well, at least for the doctors, until the expenditures for Medicare Part B began rising at alarming rates.

In an effort to stem the rising tide of physician expenditures, Congress enacted a new payment system known as the Resource-Based Relative Value Scale (RBRVS). This system was phased in over a four-year period and was designed to recognize the differences in physician specialties and to reimburse physicians according to the skill and time involved in the care that they deliver. The RBRVS reimbursement system is based on the following factors:

- A nationally uniform **relative value unit** for each service (primary care, surgical or nonsurgical)

- A geographical adjustment factor (recognizes different markets: urban or rural)

- A nationally uniform conversion factor for calculating payments (a certain dollar amount multiplied by the relative value unit)

The relative value units for each service reflect the resources involved in providing the three components of the doctor's service:

- Work (skill and effort required)

- Practice expenses (rent, staff salaries, supplies and so on)

- The cost of malpractice insurance (annual premium)

For example, if a primary care physician visit for an established patient has a relative value of 1.5 units, and the conversion factor is $37, the Medicare-approved amount is 37×1.5 or $55.50. Medicare pays 80 percent of this amount, or $44.40, and you are responsible for your 20 percent copayment of $11.10.

Recent changes in Medicare regulations protect Medicare beneficiaries from physician charges in excess of the Medicare billing limits. This regulation applies to all physicians who do not accept Medicare assignment. Nonparticipating physicians, those who do not accept assignment, engage in a practice known as balance billing, or collecting the difference between the Medicare-approved amount and their actual charge. This means that you are responsible not only for your 20 percent copayment but also for any balance above this amount. Balance billing costs Medicare beneficiaries billions of dollars in out-of-pocket expenses.

For example, if the approved charge for a specific procedure is $180, the most a nonparticipating physician may charge you is $196.65. Because nonparticipating doctors are paid 95 percent of the Medicare-approved amount and may charge 115 percent above this amount, a nonparticipating physician whose regular charge for this procedure is $275 would be allowed to collect only $196.65 ($180 × 95 percent × 115 percent). Your total out-of-pocket expense would be $52.65, which includes your copayment of $36 (20 percent of $180) plus the $16.65 in excess charge above the Medicare-approved amount.

Filing a Claim: Filing a Medicare Part B claim is much easier thanks to a change in Medicare legislation. It is now the responsibility of your doctor or medical supplier (equipment or medical supplies) to prepare and submit your Medicare claims for you. This means the following:

- Your doctor or medical supply company must file the claim even if neither of them accepts Medicare assignment.

- You cannot be charged extra for this service.

- You are responsible for paying the bill in full if the provider does not accept assignment. You will be reimbursed by Medicare.

- You should contact the Medicare carrier for your state if any provider refuses to prepare and submit your claim.

- You will still need to submit a claim with your Medicare supplemental insurer in order to collect the 20 percent copayment that is your responsibility.

We strongly recommend that you contact the Medicare carrier for your state if you encounter a problem with this system. (See appendix A.)

Medical Necessity Determinations: Physician services under Medicare are reviewed just like other services. Actual and proposed operations are reviewed most stringently. If payment is denied to the physician on the grounds that the operation was unnecessary, you are protected from having to pay for it because you could not have been expected to know this at the time.

Hospital Outpatient Services

Medicare Part B covers hospital outpatient services related to the diagnosis and treatment of an illness or injury. As with all services covered by Medicare, they must be medically necessary. These services may include, but are not limited to, diagnostic procedures (x-rays, ultrasounds, laboratory tests, endoscopic procedures and the like), therapeutic procedures (such as IV medications and physical therapy) or surgery (for example, cataract surgery or hernia repair).

Limitations on Services: Any medical service that is not medically necessary is not covered by Medicare. This includes procedures done for purely cosmetic reasons and those performed without a specific diagnosis.

Cost-Sharing: Ordinarily, when you receive services under Medicare Part B, you are responsible for meeting the annual deductible and a co-payment based on 20 percent of the Medicare-approved amount. Unfortunately, this isn't the case with hospital outpatient services.

When Congress approved the shift of some 1,400 procedures from inpatient to outpatient care, it also established a fee schedule for these procedures. Nervous hospital administrators complained that the fee schedule was unfair since their overhead and operating expenses were greater than those of doctors' offices or ambulatory care centers. As a result, Medicare pays hospitals 80 percent of their *costs,* as opposed to 80 percent of the approved fee schedule, while beneficiaries pay 20 percent of hospital *charges*. All this means that some Medicare beneficiaries pay more for a procedure when it's performed in a hospital outpatient department than if it's performed in a doctor's office or ambulatory care center, where fee limits apply. In actuality, beneficiaries are paying more than 50 percent of the cost of these services because of a loophole in the law.

How Payment Is Made: Medicare reimburses hospitals based on what it *costs* them to perform procedures, and you are responsible for 20 percent of what hospitals *charge* for these procedures. If you think there is something strange about this payment scheme, you are not alone. Unfortunately, Medicare beneficiaries have become the unintended victims of a good idea gone awry.

Medical Necessity Determinations: Outpatient services under Medicare are reviewed just like other services. Proposed operations are reviewed most stringently. If payment is denied to the physician on the grounds that the operation was unnecessary, you are protected from having to pay for it because you could not have been expected to know this at the time.

If you disagree with a decision made by your physician or Medicare+Choice plan, you have the right to appeal to either the PRO or the plan itself.

Blood Services

You are entitled to blood as medically necessary under Part B of Medicare, although you must pay the one-time blood deductible before your coverage begins. You are responsible for the cost of the first three pints of blood and then 20 percent of the Medicare-approved charge for any additional pints.

To meet the deductible, you must either pay for the blood or have it replaced. You are considered to have replaced it if an acceptable donor offers to replace it on your behalf, whether the provider or its blood supplier accepts the offer. Any portion of the deductible met during the year, either under Part A or B, counts toward the total deductible. Coverage under Part B doesn't begin until you meet your $100 deductible.

Immunosuppressive Drugs

Medicare beneficiaries who undergo a major organ transplant (heart, liver, kidneys or lungs) require powerful medications to prevent the body's immune system from rejecting the new organ. These drugs are called "immunosuppressives" because they suppress the normal action of the immune system, which is to attack invading microbes or transplanted organs. They prevent the immune system from damaging the new organ or causing damage to adjacent tissue. Medicare covers the costs of these drugs, as medically necessary, for a period of up to one year.

Summing Up

As you have seen, Medicare covers quite a bit. The problem is with the limitations on the amount of services you can receive, the requirements for receiving them and the copayments and deductibles. For Part B, for example, Medicare beneficiaries pay about 40 percent of the actual bill, not the 20 percent that Congress had intended. It should be clear to you that insurance to supplement Medicare would be nice to have; we discuss that in chapter 4.

In this chapter you will learn: The role of Medicare supplemental insurance ■ Why you need supplemental insurance ■ What the ten standard Medigap policies cover ■ How to compare supplemental policies and what to look for ■ Shopping tips to help you select the right policy ■ How and why to check the product of insurance companies ■ How to provide for nursing home coverage that Medicare doesn't

4. How to Pay for What Medicare Doesn't Cover

Medicare, as we've noted in other chapters, is an exercise in ambivalence. Congress wanted protection for senior citizens but did not want anything resembling national health insurance. It wanted to keep costs down and to give the American Medical Association and the hospitals everything they wanted. It wanted cost-sharing by beneficiaries and wanted to sharply reduce the 15 percent of their income that the elderly were spending on health care.

If this last desire is taken as the standard, Medicare is a failure. Senior citizens still spend 15 percent of their income on health care, and that proportion will rise sharply over the next few years if cost trends for the under-65 population are any indication. On the other hand, Medicare has increased access to health care for the elderly and eliminated many of the abuses found in the old systems of charity care. (It all but eliminated charity care in the process, leaving us with other problems, but that's another story.)

The dream of having guaranteed health care for Americans over age 65, supplemented by modest amounts out of their own pockets, has not been realized. What this means, in practical terms, is that you have to buy insurance to supplement Medicare if you want the degree of protection that the original program was supposed to give you. This chapter is about how to buy the best insurance for the least money.

It's not easy. Elderly Americans will spend more than $25 billion on Medicare supplemental insurance this year—an average of $900 each. If you've ever purchased supplemental insurance, you're well aware of the hodgepodge of policies that are on the market. Before there were policy standards, Medicare beneficiaries were at the mercy of insurance companies that used unscrupulous sales tactics. This led to beneficiaries purchasing policies with very little coverage or committing the larger mistake of having too many policies. Supplemental policy standards were developed by the National Association of Insurance Commissioners to help consumers compare policies and also to protect them from purchasing duplicate coverage. A complete listing of all standardized policies can be found in appendix B.

Some Insurance Concepts

Insurance is, from your angle, a gamble. Some religious groups object to it on that basis. The insurance company is betting that you will stay relatively healthy. If you do, the premiums you pay while you are insured will at least equal your actual costs of medical care, plus the costs of running the company, plus a prudent reserve for unforeseen circumstances, plus a profit. If the company is a privately held, or stock, company, the profit is distributed to the owners or shareholders or is reinvested. If it is a mutual company, the profits are returned to the members (invisibly, in the form of low premiums, or visibly, in the form of dividends or rebates). This is a little bit of an oversimplification but enough to give the flavor.

You, on the other hand, are betting that you will get sick and that the company will have to pay much more to doctors and hospitals than you put in. (If you weren't making this bet and didn't believe this would happen, you would be better off to start a savings account for future medical bills. There would be no advantage to buying insurance. In fact, this is part of the reasoning that led Medicare to experiment with medical savings accounts [MSAs]. Beneficiaries may deposit up to $6,000 in an account and use it to pay their medical expenses. In addition, they get a tax deduction for the funds contributed to the MSA.)

Insurance can also be looked at as **risk pooling**, a process whereby *all* the insured cover the expenses that only a *few* of them have in any given year. (For example, depending on the age-group, 12 to 20 percent of a population has a hospital stay in a given year. This leaves the hospital insurance premiums of the other 80 to 88 percent to cover the costs.) In practice, there's more to it than this. Insurance companies, particularly health insurers, do a great variety of things such as contracting with hospitals for guaranteed rates, fixing fee schedules for doctors, reviewing use of hospitalization and surgery and so on. But what we've told you is the essence.

Insurance companies engage in awesome statistical exercises to make sure that the claims that are paid stay in line with the premiums that are paid in. One of the insights that emerges is that protection against *all* risks is too expensive for any insurance company to offer. So all policies have *exclusions,* most have *deductibles,* many have *benefit maximums,* and a great number have a sliding scale of premiums based on the amount of risk the insured is willing to assume. Since most claims under most types of insurance are small, an insured person's willingness to assume a small risk (for example, a deductible of $200 rather than $100) is worth far more to the insurer than high-end limitations. Assuming an additional risk of $100 at the low end is worth far more to the company than reducing the maximum amount paid from $1 million to $999,900.

Total coverage for all hazards is too expensive to offer. What happens instead is bargaining between the insured and the insurance company. This takes the form of the insured person's picking and choosing among high-option plans, low-option plans and everything in between, adjusting the amount of risk the insured person is willing to assume versus the premium he has to pay until satisfied.

So goes the theory, anyway. In fact, there are pitfalls to buying insurance. The greatest of them is not knowing what it is that you want to buy in the way of protection, which is what insurance is all about.

Why You Need Supplemental Insurance

Insurance sounds like a good thing, but all is not rosy. There has been a persistent tendency in the health insurance industry to insure people against the things most can perfectly well afford—such as the $100 Medicare Part B deductible or a copayment of more than $5 per prescription under an employer's health benefit plan—and not to insure them against what they can't afford. Since the latter is the whole purpose of insurance, something is wrong.

A quick look at the Medicare chart in chapter 2 shows that gaps exist in the program. Part A, hospital insurance, requires that you pay a one-day deductible of several hundred dollars. If you should be unlucky enough to have an extended hospital stay, you then encounter daily copayments beginning on your 61st day.

Should you remain in a skilled nursing facility for more than 20 days, you incur daily copayments from the 21st through the 100th day. Even a relatively short stay could end up costing you several thousand dollars in out-of-pocket expenses.

Part B also has a deductible and a 20 percent copayment for physician and outpatient services. Since there is no limit on Part B expenses, you could find yourself facing large out-of-pocket payments. In addition, there's no coverage for prescription medications, routine dental care or routine eye examinations and corrective lenses.

These gaps clearly indicate the need for some type of insurance to supplement your Medicare coverage.

Buying Insurance to Supplement Medicare

You are not alone if you fear being bankrupted by health care costs. Knowing the facts in order to carefully evaluate and select the right Medicare supplemental policy will go far in alleviating that fear.

Our *first* assumption is that you want to protect your resources and stay out of debt. We also assume that you want to spend as little of your income as possible on health care. This means that you want to minimize your potential out-of-pocket expense. Our third assumption is that like most people, you are a little bit frightened of the cost of health care and want to buy some peace of mind as well as some insurance.

There are generally five main types of insurance plans that may be used to supplement Medicare coverage: indemnity benefit policies, employee or retiree health insurance policies, specific illness insurance policies, long-term-care insurance and Medicare supplemental policies, which include Medicare SELECT. (For more information, pick up a copy of *Guide to Health Insurance for People With Medicare* [HCFA publication 02110], available at any Social Security office.)

Of these options, only supplemental Medicare, or Medigap, policies are recognized as *certified* Medicare supplemental policies. The difference between certified policies and other forms of supplemental insurance is that certified policies are standardized. Insurance companies are permitted to market 10 standardized supplemental policies (identified as Plans A through J; see appendix B), one of which must be a core policy with basic benefits. In addition, the companies are permitted to market up to nine other plans that offer more benefits than the basic package. Some of these benefits include coverage of the Part A deductible, Part B deductible, prescription medications and excess doctor charges.

What this means is that you can compare certified policies on the basis of their premiums and select the one that offers the best value for your dollar. For example, if you decide that Plan C is the policy you want, you can get price quotes from several different insurance companies on the plan. The coverage is identical; only the price will vary. There's also a requirement designed to prevent duplication of coverage.

The Secretary of the Department of Health and Human Services certifies insurance policies as meeting the standards for Medicare supplemental insurance. Companies may not claim that their policies are certified unless they have complied with all of the underwriting requirements. The National Association of Insurance Commissioners was responsible for developing the minimum standards that must be met by all supplemental policies. We suggest that you check with your state insurance department if you have any questions concerning the status of a policy.

Traditional Insurance Policies

Now let's look at the five main types of insurance policies—including certified Medicare supplemental policies—in more detail.

- *Indemnity benefit policies* provide a fixed amount per day or per service. Usually the policy states the amount as something like "$532 per day or actual charges, whichever is lower." A policy that has high maximum payments relative to actual costs may *look* like it "covers everything," but the language of the policy, not one or two experiences with it, should be looked into.

  Indemnity policies also cover services provided by doctors, and the reimbursement is usually based on a fee schedule. Generally, the fee schedule is the most the policy will reimburse. For example, there may be a $500 maximum reimbursement for setting a broken bone.

- *Employee or retiree health insurance policies,* or health insurance policies for Medicare beneficiaries who work after age 65, usually pay for all or most of a defined set of services. They look like service benefit plans (which generally pay all the costs of a "service" such as hospitalization, surgery, outpatient care and the like) with low out-of-pocket costs to those enrolled. Since Medicare has become the *secondary* payer for plans covering employees over age 65, they have gotten somewhat less generous. (Pick up a copy of *Medicare and Other Health Benefits: Who Pays First?* [HCFA publication 02195], available at any Social Security office.) One of the possibilities offered by these plans may be a health maintenance organization (HMO) option. Be aware that there are problems associated with rejecting your employer's health plan if you are older than 65 and continue working. In that case the employer cannot offer you a plan that is the equivalent of a Medigap policy. It can pay only for the services that Medicare does not cover at all.

■ *Specific illness insurance policies* are, as the name implies, limited in their coverage. You may see these advertised as covering cancer, heart disease, accidents and so forth. You may also see individual policies covering dental care and prescription drugs, although these two types of insurance are usually sold as group policies. We generally can't recommend limited coverage insurance policies as the best method for closing the gaps in Medicare.

■ *Long-term-care insurance policies* can be used to supplement the limited nursing home coverage provided by Medicare. However, the premiums for long-term-care policies can be expensive. Some of these policies may also require prior hospitalization before paying benefits. A good long-term-care policy should cover all levels of nursing home care, and benefits should be payable beginning the first day that you require services. These policies should also cover home health care and various forms of adult day care in order to give you some flexibility in selecting the services you need. (See chapter 7 for more information on Medicare and nursing home coverage.)

■ *Medicare supplemental policies* are designed to fill in the gaps in Medicare such as the Parts A and B deductibles and copayments. These policies are coordinated with Medicare and do not duplicate Medicare coverage. All insurance companies that sell supplemental policies must comply with the federal standards for supplemental insurance. Companies are required to offer a core component of basic coverage; in addition, they may offer up to nine other plans with expanded coverage.

■ *Medicare SELECT* is a type of certified Medigap insurance policy that pays full supplemental benefits only if covered services are provided by selected providers and facilities (except in emergencies). Insurers, including some HMOs, offer Medicare SELECT in the same way standard Medigap insurance is offered. The policies meet federal standards for Medigap insurance and are regulated by the states in which they are approved. Medicare SELECT policies have lower premiums than comparable Medigap policies that do not have this selected-provider feature.

Medicare SELECT is approved for sale in all 50 states; however, it may not be offered by every insurance company or HMO. Your state insurance department can tell you if Medicare SELECT is available where you live.

Stop, Think and Decide

You'll recall that our criteria for Medicare supplemental insurance were as follows:

- To protect your assets and keep you out of debt

- To reduce your out-of-pocket expenses as much as possible

- To give you peace of mind

Using these criteria, we can screen the types of insurance policies available to supplement Medicare.

We suggest that at a minimum, you purchase a policy that covers all the deductibles and copayments for hospital and doctor bills. This means that you will have to pay only what Medicare does not reimburse the provider for, and it limits your expense to relatively minor items (with the exception of nursing home care). To protect yourself from this expense, the policy should also cover the skilled nursing facility copayment for days 21 through 100. You should also look for policies that cover physician charges in excess of the Medicare-approved charge. Policies that cover these expenses should pay at least 80 percent of the excess fee up to the full balance billing limits for nonparticipating doctors. This offers you further protection from large out-of-pocket expenses, which already cost Medicare beneficiaries billions of dollars each year.

The only way to protect yourself against excess fees is to always use a participating physician; however, we recognize that this is not always possible. Contact your nearest Social Security office and ask for a directory of doctors who accept assignment. Another way to avoid excess fees is to negotiate with the nonparticipating physician and ask him to accept the Medicare-approved payment (see chapter 5).

Here are some insurance policy features to look for:

- Guaranteed renewability

- No more than a six-month exclusion for preexisting conditions

- No limitations to single diseases such as cancer

- Payment for services in full, rather than a fixed amount such as $20 a day

- No waiting periods for coverage

The first thing that's clear is that indemnity benefit policies are unlikely to meet your needs. They pay limited benefits and would not cover the Medicare deductibles or copayments. They may also provide no additional protection on the outpatient side, which is where you need it more and more. This leaves Medigap plans (including Medicare SELECT), employee or retiree health plans, specific illness policies and long-term-care policies.

Of these options, we believe *you should keep any employer plan that you have.* It may require a small contribution, but these plans were modeled after employee plans in more generous days, and companies haven't gotten around to cutting them substantially yet. With rare exceptions, they are as good as high-option Medigap policies and possibly better. Further, a number of court cases have severely limited the right of companies to reduce benefits once you have retired, and Congress has just modified the federal bankruptcy laws so that employers' obligations to retiree medical and life insurance plans can no longer be discharged in bankruptcy proceedings. The company *must* pay. (But, of course, it cannot do so if it genuinely has no assets left.) With your employer plan, you should, of course, make sure that you are enrolled in Part A of Medicare (hospital insurance) when you turn 65. You should also purchase Part B (doctor insurance). Why? First, if you don't purchase it during your **individual enrollment period**, you have to wait until the next general enrollment period and pay an additional 10 percent premium for every year you wait. Second, enrolling keeps down the cost to your employer and helps to preserve the benefits of your plan. Third, if you don't enroll in Part B, your employer may not be able to offer you a plan that supplements Medicare. (For these reasons many companies require their retirees and employees 65 years of age and older to enroll in Part B.)

If you don't have employer-provided retiree health insurance or it is a wholly unsatisfactory plan, we recommend that you purchase either a Medigap plan or possibly Medicare SELECT.

This is the point where we have to tell you what *not* to do.

- *Do not* purchase limited-purpose insurance such as cancer insurance, accident insurance and so on. Benefits in these policies are limited to certain diagnoses, they are generally full of other limitations, and many are simply fraudulent, designed never to pay off.

- *Do not* buy a policy that excludes preexisting conditions, if at all possible. If you do, make sure that the exclusion is limited to six months at most. Federal law prevents any company from calling any policy that excludes preexisting conditions for more than six months a Medicare supplement. The fact that this is against the law doesn't mean that it won't be done, of course. Buying a policy that excludes coverage of your condition is like buying no insurance at all.

- *Do not* buy a policy that duplicates one you already have. Medicare supplemental insurance standards prohibit an insurer from selling a policy that substantially duplicates existing coverage.

- *Do not*—we hate to have to say—buy a policy just because it is endorsed by a famous figure. The endorser's chief reason for endorsing the policy is the money he gets for doing it. Policies that are advertised this way are not necessarily bad. Neither are they necessarily good.

- *Do not* buy a policy advertised with television spots and magazine ads that claim you'll face bankruptcy if you don't buy it. This is not necessarily true of insurance in general and is certainly not true of any one policy.

- *Do not* buy a policy by mail unless you know that the company is licensed to sell policies in your state. Buy a policy through the mail *only* if you are sure that it is the best. Before you buy, call or write the company and see if there is an office or agent near you. If so, deal with that office directly.

- *Do not* buy a policy that has dollar limits on total annual payments or payments over your lifetime unless those limits are *reasonably* high. Some insurance policies (but not certified supplemental policies) pay less than the Medicare-approved amounts for hospital outpatient services and services provided in a doctor's office.

- *Do not* purchase a nonrenewable policy, one that has unduly restrictive renewal clauses.

- *Do not* replace existing coverage without careful consideration of the advantages and disadvantages of both policies.

- *Do not* buy a policy just because it claims to pay for reductions in Medicare payments due to any congressionally mandated balanced budget law. The Medicare law relieves beneficiaries of responsibility for paying for the reductions in payments to providers. You'll be paying for something Medicare already provides if you fall for this one.

Some do's:

- *Do* make sure that the company that sells the policy is licensed in your state.

- *Do* check the rating of the company in *Best's Insurance Reports Life/Health,* which is available in most public libraries. This gives you an objective rating of the merits of the company and its policies.

- *Do* make sure that you know exactly what your premium is and exactly what it covers. The fact that a company offers a feature does not necessarily mean that it is included in your premium—it may cost extra. Get a complete schedule of benefits, and ask the salesperson to mark the benefits your premium covers.

- *Do* pay by check, made out to the company, not the salesperson. This gives you proof that you paid, in the form of a canceled check, and keeps the salesperson from pocketing your payment.

- *Do* take advantage of any "free look" provisions mandated by the laws of your state. These allow you to buy a policy and cancel it with no obligation within a certain period if you decide that it is not what you want.

- *Do* ask the salesperson or agent for information on the average out-of-pocket expenses for holders of the policy. This will tell you how much protection you really are buying.

- *Do* look very carefully at the coverage offered for doctors' fees over and above the Medicare-approved charge. A policy that covers only your 20 percent copayment is better than nothing, but you are still responsible for the fee up to the balance billing limit.

- *Do* look for a policy that covers prescription drug charges. Prescription drug coverage is relatively expensive. Studies on older people have shown that they spend either a relatively small amount on prescription drugs or a lot.

- *Do* call your state insurance department and make sure that the policy is approved by them before you buy. (Approval to sell a policy in a state does not mean that it is a good one, simply that it violates none of the laws and conditions on insurance in that state.)

- *Do* make sure the policy you select is automatically adjusted to cover increases in Medicare's copayments and deductibles.

You can use the form on page 106 to check your policy against our recommendations.

Filing Claims for Supplemental Insurance

One of the things you have to face with traditional insurance companies, and occasionally with managed care plans, is filing a claim. At one time Medicare beneficiaries had to complete and submit their own claims for Part B services if their physician did not accept assignment. However, that has changed for the better now that physicians are required by law to complete and submit claims for Part B services. This means less paperwork for you; however, if you want to be reimbursed for your 20 percent copayment, you still need to file a claim with your Medigap insurance carrier.

It's important that your physician file the claim within a reasonable period of time; otherwise, you'll be delayed in filing your Medigap insurance claim. Some Medigap insurers require that you enclose a copy of your Medicare Summary Notice (MSN) before you file a claim, and you won't get an MSN until the claim is filed and processed by the carrier. (See the sample form on pages 78-79.)

There is, however, a downside to this policy that could cause a few problems. If your physician does not accept assignment, she may request full payment at the time services are delivered. This may mean a rather hefty out-of-pocket expense for which you may not be reimbursed by Medicare for a number of months. In addition, without an MSN you won't be able to file a claim with your Medigap insurance, which means a further delay in getting your money.

If you do not get the amount you believe the policy should pay, or if the insurer rejects the claim, see chapter 8, which is a troubleshooting kit for all sorts of situations. The one thing you should know before you go into a full-scale effort is that insurers often reject claims *because they're duplicates*. We believe that insurers would be well advised to simply notify you that the claim is a duplicate and that processing of the original is still going on, rather than telling you it has been rejected. But that day has not yet arrived.

MEDICARE SUPPLEMENTAL
INSURANCE COMPARISON WORKSHEET

Use the information provided by the insurance companies to complete this worksheet.

Company Name	Policy 1	Policy 2	Policy 3	Policy 4
Policy/Plan Name				
Premium: May be affected by age and sex				
Monthly	$	$	$	$
Quarterly	$	$	$	$
Semiannually	$	$	$	$
Annually	$	$	$	$
Does the supplemental policy cover the deductibles and copayments listed below?	If so, place a checkmark in the appropriate column for each policy.			
Medicare Part A: Hospital				
Initial deductible* $				
61st to 90th Day Copayment* $ /day				
91st to 150th Day Copayment* $ /day				
100% of Medicare-approved expenses for additional 365 days				
Skilled Nursing Care 21st to 100th Day Copayment* $ /day				
Medicare Part B: Physician				
Initial deductible $100				
20% Copayment				
Does the supplemental policy provide any additional benefits?	If so, place a checkmark in the appropriate column for each policy.			
Prescription drugs				
Private duty nursing				
Additional physicians' fees				
Skilled Nursing Care				
Number of days available	___	___	___	___
Preventive services				
Emergency services (travel)				

*Fill in amounts from current benefit year.

In this chapter you will learn: Why it's important to negotiate with your doctor ▪ When to negotiate with your doctor ▪ How assignment can save you money ▪ How the balance billing limits can save you money ▪ What is meant by fully informing a patient ▪ How to get the right diagnosis ▪ When to get a second opinion ▪ How to use advance directives

5. Negotiating With Your Doctor

The image that comes to mind when people think of negotiating is usually confrontational: strikes and diplomatic encounters. They also think that the term implies that something has gone wrong, and the negotiating is being done to set it right. People also think in terms of winners and losers. The word—at least as defined by good ol' *Webster's*—doesn't have the connotations of confrontation, things going awry and wins and losses. Negotiation simply means "the carrying on of business" or "dealing with some matter that requires ability for its successful handling."

It's fair to say that there is a confrontation of sorts going on between many members of the medical profession and American society, that it's happening because things have gone wrong and that there will be winners and losers. But that doesn't have to be the case in your dealings with doctors. We make no secret of the fact that if it does come down to a win/lose situation, we prefer the consumer, the patient—you—to be the winner. But often the discussions that we suggest in this chapter can be carried out so that you *and* the doctor win.

Of course, a win-win situation depends on what each party views as a successful outcome. Let's use accepting assignment as an example. If you use a doctor who does not currently accept assignment and you persuade her to accept it in your case (the best outcome) or at least for the treatment of the moment (better than nothing), she is giving up the right to charge you more than 20 percent of the Medicare-approved price. She is also required by law to file your Part B claim for you. She may consider this a loss; that is fine. How she looks at it is up to her. In any case, negotiating shouldn't be an exercise in doctor bashing. Think of it, rather, as helping your doctor to help you as much as she can and educating her about the medical marketplace. Negotiating is getting the best service for the best price.

It has been said that "the man (or woman) who asks for nothing is quite likely to get it." To negotiate successfully, you have to know what you're trying to get. We specify some goals for you in this chapter. You should aim for the following:

- Paying no more than the Medicare-approved charge for the services you receive

- Getting the best possible treatment to produce what you consider the best overall outcome

- Staying in control of your treatment—being able to make and enforce the choices that you think are best for you and avoiding unnecessary risk and expense—at all times—even if you are unable to communicate your wishes

For each of these issues, we give you the background you need to deal with the issue, some suggestions for dealing with the general situation and some examples (or scenarios) of successful negotiations.

Why It's Hard to Negotiate With Doctors

Nurses (among others) have a longstanding joke that the initials M.D. stand for "mostly divine." With divine beings, one does not negotiate. One prays. It is not surprising, therefore, that the idea of negotiating with a doctor is foreign to most people.

It should not be foreign. It should be standard practice. There are a number of reasons why it isn't. At a time when doctors were among the few educated people in society—when only about 4 percent of the population had a college education and most adults had not finished high school—it was unrealistic to expect that the patient could understand matters well enough to negotiate treatment without a crash course in biology. Rather than provide it, doctors relied on intimidation, fueled by their extremely rare level of learning and high social position, to get patients to cooperate. This has always been the style of physicians in largely unlettered societies. In the late nineteenth century, the style of modern medicine was struggling to establish itself as the only "scientific" kind of medicine and to end legislative control of medicine and establish control by the profession. This effort reinforced the tendency to treat the patient as a child—a sick child, at that.

Another reason has its roots in the history of American medicine. In the nineteenth century, the group of medical practitioners who had the M.D. degree—only one of the kinds of degrees, or certificates of study, issued to the various types of medical practitioners—made a move to take over all of medical practice through the legislatures. This was done at a time when those with the M.D. degree, who practiced a kind of medicine that is called "allopathic," had no greater claim to a scientific foundation for their practices than any of the other schools did. (Those other schools, for example, practiced osteopathic, chiropractic, naturopathic and homeopathic brands of medicine. They still survive.)

Part of the strategy for taking over the whole medical field was a conscious, long-range effort to place holders of the M.D. degree (as opposed to other kinds of doctors such as osteopaths) on a pedestal. The strategy required a "mythology of medicine"—a presentation of M.D.-style medicine as far more scientific and far more founded in careful, controlled experiments than it really was (or, for that matter, far more than it is today). Doctors are still trained in the mythology. The game still goes on. A federal court concluded that the American Medical Association (AMA) had deliberately engaged in an attempt to restrain the practices of chiropractors.

Medicine has much in common with engineering. The engineer solves problems by trying out solutions, based on general knowledge of a problem, until something works. If she's good, it works on the first try. If not, she keeps trying. Medicine has little in common with the hard sciences such as physics, in which the classic experiments work all of the time.

Finally, some doctors consciously and subconsciously cultivate an aloofness, an above-the-fray attitude and a hypercompetent appearance. To some extent this is a matter of emotional survival. But this attitude is acknowledged by many to get in the way of sympathizing with patients' personal concerns about illness, growing old and death.

With these factors still dominant in medical training and practice, it's up to the patient—you—to educate doctors to treat you as you wish to be treated.

Why It's Important   Medicare beneficiaries—whether over 65 or disabled—need to negotiate more than most people do. There are several reasons for this:

- Most Americans experience their first serious illnesses only when they are about age 50 or older. (People may have heart attacks in their 30s, but longer-term illnesses, for most people, come with age.) Because of this, the most expensive illnesses come when people have reduced incomes, are not fully employed and are dependent on Medicare for health coverage.

- Medicare pays most of the hospital expenses of the elderly, but the proportion of nonhospital expenses covered is falling rapidly. This is happening at a time when care is increasingly being shifted out of the hospital into other settings. Medicare was designed largely as hospital insurance and has not caught up with the reality of current medical practice.

- Almost no form of supplemental insurance covers everything that the elderly need.

- The cost of treatment, the physical and psychological burdens of treatment and the effect on relatives are all determined mostly by the doctor.

If you want to have *any* influence on the cost of your treatment, how much (or little) you benefit from it and how and when you go, you have to negotiate with doctors. There's no other option.

There are three more reasons to take this business of negotiating seriously. First, doctors in many areas are hungry for patients right now and getting hungrier. The United States is heading toward a ratio of two doctors per 1,000 people, while there is good evidence that 1.2 to 1.4 per 1,000 is what is really needed. From the patient's side, the doctor glut shows up in increased exposure to treatments designed to augment the doctor's income rather than the patient's health. From the doctor's side, it means a scramble for a static pool of patients. It means that the loss of a single patient is more serious and that more effort needs to be made to keep patients happy. There are still regions of the country where one or two doctors monopolize a specialty, but they are becoming fewer.

Second, the new breed of doctors—the most recent graduates of medical school—are much more inclined to involve patients in treatment decisions than their older colleagues are. Part of the reason for this is dissatisfaction with the traditional style of practice. Another reason is the knowledge that fully informing patients (or doing what they *think* is fully informing patients) protects them to some degree from malpractice suits—they can blame a poor outcome partly on the patient's dumb choice. You can take advantage of their sincere desire to inform you to get better care at a better price.

Third, when one enters a large hospital with lots of departments and lots of specialties—particularly a teaching hospital—several doctors are likely to be involved in the patient's care. The admitting physician may shrink into the background as surgeons, radiologists, nuclear medicine specialists, internists, cardiologists, pulmonary medicine specialists, intensivists and a corps of residents and doctors get into the act. Often no one person is clearly in charge. Some doctors and hospitals realize the danger (to patients and to their malpractice insurer) in this situation and are trying to do something about it, but those efforts are in their infancy. It may well be that if you want anyone to be in charge, it will have to be you. Thus, it is essential that you and someone you trust be prepared to negotiate your care.

The First Big Issue: Prices

We said that throughout this book we give you bits of the history of the Medicare program and just enough technical detail to make you an empowered consumer, but not enough to overwhelm you. The first big issue is prices. Talking about prices in Medicare requires, first and foremost, that we talk about assignment. Assignment is defined as the transfer of benefits of a policy to another party; for example, telling your insurance company to send the check directly to your doctor or hospital rather than to you.

Assignment is one of those topics that has a long, complicated history and deserves a bit of background information. When a doctor agrees to take assignment, she agrees to accept the payment that the Medicare carrier has decided is appropriate for the service she rendered. This does not mean you pay nothing; Medicare pays 80 percent, and you (or your insurance company) pay 20 percent. The Medicare check goes to her. You have to deal only with your portion of the bill and with your supplemental insurance company, if you have one. If you have insurance that covers the 20 percent that Medicare doesn't pay (called the copayment), you pay nothing. If you don't have supplemental insurance, then the 20 percent copayment is an out-of-pocket expense for you. That is why it's important to carry supplemental insurance.

Until recently, doctors could pick and choose whether or not to take assignment on a service-by-service basis. Now they are either participating doctors, which means that they take assignment on all services they render, or nonparticipating, which means that they can still pick and choose among patients and services, taking assignment on some but not on others.

Doctors and Their Prices: History Past and Present

The Code of Hammurabi, a compilation of Babylonian law that dates to 1750 B.C.—almost 40 centuries ago—sets limits on how much doctors may charge. (It also prescribes strict punishment for bad results of treatment.) Some 140 years before the American Revolution, the colony of Virginia set maximum allowable prices for doctors' services. As you can imagine, control of doctors' fees has been a big issue with the medical profession from the time it first recognized itself as such.

Doctors in the United States have argued strongly with everyone who has tried to limit fees in some way. When health insurance became generally available because of employer funding after World War II, health insurers faced a dilemma. They had to get doctors to accept enough payment from them to convince the insured that expenses really were covered. They had to make the amount small enough that policies were affordable. The result was the usual, customary and reasonable reimbursement system.

Why Assignment and Participation Are Important Issues for You

The importance of assignment and participation can best be explained by examples. Suppose you have a cardiac catheterization. (This is a procedure in which a small tube is inserted into the arteries of the heart, or into the heart itself, for diagnosis and sometimes treatment. Dye can be injected to show the arteries and detect blockages, arteries can be dilated with a balloon, and drugs can be injected to abort heart attacks.) The doctor charges $3,000. He is free to pull this number out of his hat; there are no set prices. It may be much more, or much less, than his colleagues charge. Most studies show that at least a 2-to-1 ratio can be found in a given community—that is, the highest-charging doctor charges at least twice as much as the lowest-charging. (Remember, however, that price has nothing to do with quality. High prices do not necessarily mean better care.)

If he is a participating doctor, he has agreed to accept assignment—which, again, means accepting the Medicare-approved payment as payment in full—for all services he renders to Medicare beneficiaries. (Again, this does not mean you pay nothing; Medicare pays 80 percent, and you [or your insurance company] pay 20 percent.) Does this mean that Medicare will pay 80 percent of the $3,000? No. It means that Medicare pays 80 percent of the Medicare-approved amount, which is based on the Resource-Based Relative Value Scale (RBRVS) reimbursement system.

Unlike the old usual, customary and reasonable payment system, which rewarded doctors for constantly raising their prices, the RBRVS considers the skills and resources required to deliver medical services. The RBRVS reimbursement system is based on the following factors:

- A nationally uniform relative value unit for each service (primary care, surgical or nonsurgical)

- A geographical adjustment factor (recognizes different markets: urban or rural)

- A nationally uniform conversion factor for calculating payments (a certain dollar amount multiplied by the relative value unit)

The relative value units for each service reflect the resources involved in providing the three components of the doctor's service:

- Work (skill and effort required)

- Practice expenses (rent, staff salaries, supplies and so on)

- The cost of malpractice insurance (annual premium)

Let's say the approved charge is $2,000. Medicare pays the doctor 80 percent of that—$1,600—and you or your insurance company pay the remaining 20 percent—$400. Your doctor files the claim, the check goes to him, and he bills you for the remaining $400. You pay it or file a claim with your supplemental insurance company. If you have not met your $100 annual deductible, it will be subtracted from the amount that Medicare pays. You or your insurance company pay it, depending on your policy. Both situations are illustrated in the following chart:

Example 1: Doctor Accepts Assignment

Actual charge:	$3,000
Medicare-approved charge:	$2,000
Medicare pays: 80% of $2,000 =	$1,600
You pay: $2,000 − $1,600 =	$ 400
If $100 Medicare Part B deductible not met:	
Medicare-approved charge:	$2,000
Less Part B deductible:	$ 100
Medicare pays: 80% of $2,000 (= $1,600), less $100 =	$1,500
You pay:	$ 500
Total payment to doctor:	$2,000

By becoming a Medicare-participating physician, your doctor has agreed to eat the other $1,000. It's no great loss. He knew that he wasn't going to get it anyway. That's because his charge of $3,000 is greater than the Medicare-approved amount based on the RBRVS fee schedule. As a participating physician, he knows that his reimbursement is based on the fee schedule, and he is willing to accept this amount as payment in full.

But what happens if you go to a nonparticipating doctor? In addition to the 20 percent copayment, you are also responsible for any excess charge up to the balance billing limit, which is no more than 115 percent of the Medicare-approved charge. Medicare has developed a rather complicated formula for determining how much a doctor may charge for his services. The balance billing limit is determined by multiplying the Medicare-approved amount by 95 percent and then by 115 percent. The immediate effect of this is to save you money when you must use a doctor who does not accept assignment.

Using the figures from our previous example, the doctor's charge is $3,000, the Medicare-approved amount for a nonparticipating doctor is $1,900 ($2,000 × 95 percent), and the balance billing limit is $2,185 ($1,900 × 115 percent). Medicare pays $1,520 ($1,900 × 80 percent), which leaves a balance of $665 for you and your supplemental insurance. *You are not responsible for the remaining $815.*

The doctor files the claim with Medicare, and you file a claim with your supplemental insurance carrier to collect your 20 percent. You are responsible for the difference between the Medicare-approved amount and the balance billing limit. Here's the arithmetic again:

Example 2: Doctor Does Not Accept Assignment

Actual charge:	$3,000
Medicare-approved charge: 95% of $2,000 =	$1,900
Balance billing limit: 115% of $1,900 =	$2,185
Medicare pays: 80% of $1,900 =	$1,520
You pay: $2,185 − $1,520 =	$ 665
If $100 Medicare Part B deductible not met:	
Medicare pays: 80% of $1,900 =	$1,520
Less Part B deductible:	$ 100
Medicare pays:	$1,420
You pay: $2,185 − 1,420 =	$ 765
Total payment to doctor:	$2,185

Example 3: Comparison of an Assigned Versus a Nonassigned Claim

	Doctor takes assignment	Doctor does not take assignment
Actual charge:	$3,000	$3,000
Medicare-approved charge:	$2,000	$1,900
Balance billing limit:	—	$2,185
Medicare pays:	$1,600	$1,520
You pay:	$ 400	$ 665
If Part B $100 deductible not met:		
Medicare-approved charge:	$1,600	$1,520
Less Part B deductible:	$ 100	$ 100
Medicare pays:	$1,500	$1,420
You pay:	$ 500	$ 765

The limits on balance billing will definitely save you money when you must use a nonparticipating doctor. If your doctor's charges exceed the maximum charges permitted by law, neither you nor your insurance company has to pay the difference between the maximum charge and the doctor's actual charge. However, you will be responsible for the difference between the approved charge and the balance billing limit. Follow the example shown below.

Example 4: Comparison of Out-of-Pocket Expenses With Balance Billing Limits on Nonparticipating Doctors

Actual charge:	$3,000
Medicare-approved charge:	$1,900
Balance billing limit:	$2,185
Medicare pays:	$1,520
You pay without limits:	$1,480
You pay with limits:	$ 665
You save:	$ 815

It should be obvious that persuading your doctor to take assignment on all your bills—or going to a doctor who accepts assignment—can save you large sums of money. Since most people over 65 are not particularly wealthy, the potential savings really count. You should not feel that you are cheating your doctor by asking him to accept assignment. The charge that Medicare has determined as "reasonable," in most cases, takes into account what other doctors charge. Remember, too, that the relationship of real costs to charges in all of American medicine is not tight. It is unlikely that whatever Medicare pays is below what it cost your doctor to provide the service, plus a reasonable profit. Your doctor may *feel* that the Medicare payment is too low. Unless he presents you with hard evidence that Medicare is not covering him real costs, don't worry. Point out to him that other doctors who accept assignment seem to do well.

Some New Incentives for Doctors to Accept Assignment

The States: Medical licenses are still granted by states, not by the federal government, even though proposals for a national medical license are growing more frequent. (The reasons for these demands range from evidence that many states handle the licensing of doctors in a haphazard way to the desire to have uniform disciplining of incompetent practitioners.)

Because the states have the licensing power, they can attach requirements to the license. Massachusetts became the first state to require mandatory assignment as a condition of licensure. Rhode Island passed a mandatory assignment law; however, it was not linked to licensure. Other states that took action to encourage Medicare assignment are Connecticut, Minnesota, New York, Ohio, Pennsylvania and Vermont. Pennsylvania's law bans balance billing (charging the difference between the Medicare-approved amount and what the doctor usually charges), while Connecticut's and Vermont's laws have eligibility requirements based on income.

The Federal Government: The federal government has not yet attempted to require that doctors accept assignment as a condition of being in the Medicare program. Instead, from 1980 through 1988, the Reagan administration attempted to use free market incentives to encourage greater physician participation. Some of the incentives actually do have a chance of encouraging more doctors to participate.

Some of the incentives are of direct benefit to you:

- The *Directory of Participating Doctors in Your Area* is available to you free of charge. You should receive a notice of the availability of this directory annually, and you can obtain one at any time by writing to the Medicare carrier for your state. Copies are available for review at Social Security offices. Medicare-participating doctors also can display emblems or certificates that show they accept assignment on all Medicare claims. The directory shows the specialties of the doctors as well. (A list of Medicare carriers is contained in appendix A.)

- If your hospital refers you to a doctor for outpatient care, the hospital must *inform you if the doctor is a nonparticipating doctor and must identify at least one participating doctor from whom you can obtain the same services,* if one is available.

- If a nonparticipating physician is preparing to perform **elective surgery** on you and will not take assignment, and if the charge for surgery will exceed $500, *you must be provided with written notice of the estimated actual charge, the estimated approved charge and the estimated expense to you* (or your insurance plan). This will give you time to seek the same services from a participating doctor or to negotiate with your doctor to provide the services on assignment.

There are a few additional incentives for doctors. Each Medicare Summary Notice (the paper that the Medicare carrier sends to tell you what it paid for) that contains unassigned charges includes a message reminding you that you would have fared better if you had obtained the services from a participating doctor. In addition, claims that do not require investigation by the Medicare carrier to resolve a discrepancy are paid for participating doctors about a week earlier than those for nonparticipating doctors. If a doctor has cash flow problems, this can make a big difference and can be a real incentive to become a participating doctor.

Negotiating With Your Doctor About Fees

The most effective way to negotiate fees with your doctor is with your feet: Attempt to find a doctor who is a Medicare participant. Doctors need customers these days, and the need will grow. It will be very easy, as time goes by, to find a participating doctor—even if you don't live in Connecticut, Massachusetts, Minnesota, New York, Ohio, Pennsylvania, Rhode Island or Vermont.

But there may be reasons for not using a participating doctor:

- You may not be able to find one.

- You may have been getting genuinely good service from your family doctor, who, for whatever reason, does not participate.

- A specialist your family doctor refers you to may be the only one in town—or a good one—and may not participate.

Whether or not the doctor participates, you have a reason to negotiate fees. You especially have a reason if the doctor doesn't participate because in that situation the amount you wind up paying out of pocket—or that has to be covered by your insurance—will be up to the balance billing limit. You may also decide not to use this doctor again unless he agrees to accept assignment. In other words, it is just good business to bargain.

There are other reasons for negotiating. Many doctors' prices are pulled out of thin air. They are not set by any market forces the way the prices for other services are. For most services, prices are publicly available and advertised. With doctors, it doesn't work that way, if only because the prices aren't published. If you're involved in a Medicare private fee-for-service plan (PFFSP) or a Medicare medical savings account (MSA), it becomes especially important for you to keep an eye on the price of your health care. While these plans are designed to give you more flexibility in choosing practitioners, they also place more responsibility on your shoulders to closely monitor fees.

PFFSPs use their own payment schedules that do not follow the Medicare-approved rate schedule. These plans shift more of the risk to you and away from the physician. Beneficiaries who elect to use an MSA must also monitor what they are spending for medical care. Unlike the PFFSPs, there are no limits on what providers can charge above the amount paid by the Medicare MSA plan. Failure to negotiate fees under these circumstances could result in substantial out-of-pocket expenses for you.

The Second Big Issue: Treatment

Now let's discuss negotiating with your doctor about treatment. The basic questions you should ask and discuss with your doctor are the following:

- Does she recognize her obligation to inform you fully?

- What are her criteria for the success or failure of a treatment?

- How sure is she of your diagnosis? How did she establish it?

- If she has recommended surgery, is there a medical treatment option? If she recommended medical treatment, is there a surgical option?

- If she has recommended surgery, where can you get a second opinion? What are the various surgical options?

- If she has recommended medical treatment, what are the various medical options?

- Is she willing to accept your prior instructions concerning your treatment in the event that you become incapacitated?

- If (when) she calls in specialists, how will you and she maintain control of the team treating you?

- What steps will be taken to control potentially harmful diagnostic tests?

The Doctor's Obligation to Inform You Fully

The number of situations in which it is legally permissible for a doctor not to inform you fully about your condition and the treatment options available has shrunk dramatically over the past three decades. It is safe to say that in most states the only cases in which a full explanation of your situation can legally be withheld from you are those in which your mental competence is in doubt. Standards for finding you incompetent are becoming stricter. However, this does not mean that you will, in fact, be fully informed.

Ideally, your doctor should sign the People's Medical Society Code of Practice. This is the most detailed attempt we know of to define what informed consent *ought* to mean from the patient's point of view. Unfortunately, if the number who have agreed to sign the code is any indication, most doctors don't agree with the People's Medical Society view of informed consent; you have to be on your guard. This does not mean refusing to trust your doctor. It does mean recognizing that he may have not one, but several, blinders on. Below we show the People's Medical Society Code of Practice in the form of questions you should ask your doctor:

- Does he post a printed schedule of fees for office visits, procedures, testing and surgery?

- Does he provide itemized bills?

- Is he available for nonemergency telephone consultation during certain hours each week?

- Does he schedule appointments to allow the time necessary to see you, with minimal waiting time? Will he promptly return phone calls and report test results to you?

- Will he allow and encourage you to bring a friend or relative into the examining room with you?

- Will he facilitate getting your medical and hospital records to you and provide you with copies of your test results?

- Will he let you know your prognosis, including whether or not your condition is terminal or will cause disability or pain?

- Will he explain why further diagnostic procedures or treatments are necessary?

- Will he discuss diagnostic, treatment and medication options for your particular problem with you (including the option of no treatment) and describe in understandable terms the risk of each alternative, the possibility of pain, the effect on your functioning, the number of visits each alternative would entail and the cost of each?

- Will he discuss his qualifications to perform the proposed diagnostic measures or treatments?

- Will he let you know of organizations, support groups and medical and lay publications that will assist you in understanding, monitoring and treating your problem?

- Will he agree not to proceed until you are satisfied that you understand the risks and benefits of each alternative and he has your agreement on a particular course of action?

If you ask the doctor these questions, you'll be pretty well informed about your treatment and the doctor's style of practice. But to get a serious response, you may still have to work around some obstacles that may impede communication.

First, a general prejudice exists in our society against the aged (and the disabled). There is a general prejudice against people who appear lower than middle-class in social status. Nothing in the education of a doctor necessarily removes either of these prejudices. As a Medicare beneficiary, you are (automatically) either aged or disabled. As a recipient of Social Security, you may be poor.

Second, doctors are told that they must arrange treatment according to your best interest, but that means *the doctor's* view of your best interest. Nothing in the training of doctors prepares them to be more sympathetic to your view of your own best interest than to their own. They are raised in the tradition of "doctor knows best." If you want them to treat you according to your view of your best interest, you have to tell them. Loudly. Clearly. Especially loudly.

Third, doctors in general, and American doctors in particular, don't like to treat chronic conditions. (Chronic conditions are those that are marked by long duration and frequent recurrence and are difficult or impossible to cure once and for all.) Doctors want a clear victory over disease, and they want it quickly.

Fourth, you may have difficulty in seeing, hearing or speaking. This will make communicating with you more difficult. On top of your chronic conditions, this will make you even more frustrating to the doctor, and you more frustrated with him.

Fifth, you may have dementia—the general label for a condition in which your brain is not working as well as it did at one time. It may be mild to severe, acute or chronic. It may or may not be caused by, or made worse by, drugs the doctor has prescribed for you. The problem is that once there is any sign of it, your ideas and opinions may be discounted. There is also a medical prejudice in the belief that anyone who is not a perfectly functioning adult either has a diminished pain response or doesn't mind pain. (It is only now being recognized that very small children *do* need anesthetics for surgery.) In addition, if you're uncomfortable or in pain, you will be less likely to make yourself heard.

It's up to you to make sure that you are informed enough to give consent to whatever the doctor has in mind for you. Trust in him is not enough. Liking him is not enough. Both are good, but they don't add up to *knowing* what he plans for your treatment, what alternatives are available and what might go wrong with each. *You can't count on him to overcome all the prejudices about the elderly and the disabled in our society.*

Having a friend or relative assist you in dealing with the doctor will help with the fourth and fifth points we've just made. But more important, having someone with you will keep the doctor on his toes. That means you get better care. In fact, if you feel that you are functioning at less than full capacity, or if there is some sign that the doctor believes so, we recommend that you insist on having someone with you. (Some of us may never attain what the medical profession considers "full capacity.")

With all the hurdles that have to be jumped to get to the point where you feel fully informed, some criteria are needed. We believe you can feel fully informed if (and *only* if):

- You understand what is wrong with you, what the doctor thought was wrong with you before he arrived at the current diagnosis and how he arrived at the current diagnosis.

- You understand the medical and surgical treatments available and the risks and benefits of each; the doctor should have given you some objective measure of the risks.

Let's look at an example.

For a while you've been feeling run-down and have had a vague, dull pain in your abdomen. Lately it has become much sharper, and you are having diarrhea. Going to the bathroom relieves the pain, but only for a short time. You've been taking some medicine you bought off the shelf at the drugstore, but lately it isn't working. You have started to lose weight and to have soaking sweats at night. You've been putting off going to the doctor because you're afraid he'll find cancer. But you now feel so bad that you want something done. You wisely decide to go to the doctor.

He examines you and discovers that you are bleeding slowly from somewhere in your digestive tract. He draws blood for tests and asks the laboratory (which is fortunately in the same building as his office) to get the results back to him "stat" ("right now!"). You sit in the waiting room for about an hour, with time out for a few trips to the bathroom. The nurse calls you back to the examining room. The doctor says, "You definitely have a bleeding problem somewhere inside. You're anemic, which could account for the tiredness. I was worried that you might have a tumor in the colon, but the blood tests show signs of something called inflammatory bowel disease."

He continues, "I want to do a colonoscopy on you. It's a simple procedure I can do here in the office. We place a small tube with a light and a lens into your colon through the rectum. I can take biopsies to confirm my guess and also look for tumors. If you have polyps, which could cause the bleeding, I can remove any I see. We'll sedate you lightly. All you'll have is a few cramps, and you won't remember much."

You ask what he suspects—a tumor, inflammatory bowel disease or something else. He tells you that you might have a tumor, an inflamed bowel or both or possibly a parasite causing diarrhea. You ask why he can't use x-rays and tell him that you don't like the sound of the colonoscopy.

"I could take a large bowel series," the doctor replies, "which involves an enema of barium. It's nearly as uncomfortable as the colonoscopy and doesn't differentiate between some of the conditions I think you might have. We might still wind up with a colonoscopy after the x-rays if we find polyps. I want to examine a stool specimen for parasites, but I'm pretty sure you don't have them. The other symptoms don't fit." You ask if there are any other tests that might be used. The doctor says no. It's x-rays or the colonoscopy. You ask about the risks.

The doctor says, "It's possible that I will accidentally perforate your bowel; that happens about once for every 450 colonoscopies done in the United States. My record is better. I've done 2,000 of these and only perforated the bowel in two cases. If this happens, I will have to put you in the hospital. It's almost certain that surgery will be needed. Survival for major perforations of the bowel without surgery is poor."

You ask what will happen with each of the conditions the doctor suspects. He tells you that with a benign tumor, you'll continue to be miserable; with a cancerous one, you might die. A parasitic infection might clear up or leave you growing weaker and weaker. It could be treated with drugs, but these would have no effect if there were no parasites. An attack of inflammatory bowel disease could subside on its own, or it could ultimately lead to the need for serious surgery to remove a large part of the intestines. There are fairly good drugs to treat it.

You reluctantly agree to the colonoscopy, which is a bit more unpleasant than the doctor made it sound, but not as bad as you had feared. The biopsy shows that you have a mild case of inflammatory bowel disease. The doctor prescribes medicine for the cramps and diarrhea and tells you that he is putting you on steroids.

"Like a weightlifter?" you ask in some puzzlement. The doctor tells you no, there is another kind of steroid. You ask about side effects. He tells you that there are some serious ones, but they are associated only with long-term use. He suspects that you will be off steroids in a month or two. You ask about short-term side effects. He tells you that these include weight gain, a puffy face and lowered resistance to infection. You ask if there are any others. The doctor tells you that there is something called "steroid psychosis" and that he usually puts patients who are on high doses in the hospital. He tells you that the dose he proposes for you is not high enough to worry about.

You go home, take the drug and almost immediately feel better. The diarrhea stops, the cramps go away, you stop soaking the sheets with sweat at night, and you feel even better. In fact, you feel wonderful. Then you clearly feel your heart missing beats. You call the doctor in a panic. He tells you to come to the office right away. He orders an electrocardiogram (EKG), which shows nothing seriously out of order except missed beats, and more blood tests, again "stat."

"Steroids can cause increased potassium loss in the urine," the doctor tells you. "Potassium is an element in the blood that helps control heartbeat and muscle contraction. Yours is very low. Apparently, your body reacts more strongly than most to that effect. I'll prescribe a potassium supplement for you."

You point out, with a bit of embarrassment, that the doctor mentioned nothing about heart problems when he prescribed the drug. You also ask if feeling abnormally good is another side effect. The doctor admits that these are side effects he didn't tell you about because he did not think them likely in your case. He tells you that he will reduce the dosage of steroid in a few days, and he devotes a lot of time to warning you about stomach irritation from the potassium supplement.

The point of the story is this: You'll have to work to get this much; your doctor should be able to give it to you. If he doesn't know, make him look it up. With in-office computer services for doctors now readily available, he can get the answer within seconds. Making him look up the answer will contribute to his continuing professional education, raise the general level of medical practice in the United States and, possibly, save your life.

Let's continue with our list of criteria for being a more informed consumer. We believe you can feel fully informed if (and *only* if):

- You have a clear understanding of the doctor's criteria for the success or failure of a treatment—whether or not he expects a complete recovery, and if he does not, what improvement he hopes for. (More on this later.)

- You know the best that can be expected from the treatment you are receiving for a person of your age, sex and general condition. Sometimes cures aren't possible, but it may be possible to make you much more comfortable. Doctors use the word "palliation" to describe treating a condition that can't be cured in order to make the patient more comfortable and better able to function. If you *both* understand what he's after, you will control your treatment much more effectively.

- You understand who will be in charge (you) if you are referred to a specialist and you've had a chance to make your own choice.

- You have received a second opinion from someone who is not professionally or financially associated with the doctor who recommended the surgery, if surgery is recommended.

- The doctor has disclosed any financial benefit he will receive from recommending a treatment or prescribing a drug. (The AMA code of ethics requires this, and state laws should, too.)

- You have made arrangements to ensure that your wishes are carried out if you are unable to remain in charge of your treatment.

- You brought a friend to the visit with the doctor, and he feels comfortable on the above points.

Let's look at a hypothetical example. You have had arthritis for several years but have been taking aspirin and exercising as prescribed. You have been doing well in general, and you have been free of pain and stiffness most of the time. Now, suddenly, your right knee is almost too painful to move. You increase the dosage of aspirin as your doctor instructed you, but that doesn't seem to help. You call her, and she tells you to come to the office the next day. She looks at the knee, which is hot, red and swollen.

She takes some blood for a test, suggests that you rest the knee as much as possible and splint it at night and gives you a prescription for a nonsteroidal anti-inflammatory drug (these drugs are like aspirin but much more powerful). The test results come back and show that you have rheumatoid arthritis on top of the osteoarthritis that was already damaging the knee. (Both forms of arthritis can damage joints. Rheumatoid arthritis is generally much more severe.) Various drugs for both forms of arthritis are tried without success. You develop stomach bleeding with one of the anti-inflammatory drugs and have to be put on steroids for a short while. This produces a good deal of relief, but your doctor does not want to use steroids for a long time. Finally, she recommends replacement of the knee with an artificial one. You ask why.

"You've effectively lost use of the knee," she says. "If we could get it quieted down for a while, we could work on some physical therapy and try to preserve enough function to let you at least walk. But we just can't do it. I think surgery is the only alternative." She gives you the name of an orthopedic surgeon, Konrad Kowboi, who has done numerous knee replacements.

You go to see the surgeon. He examines the knee and says he agrees that surgery is needed. He can do it on Wednesday, and he starts to ask his nurse to reserve a room for you at the hospital. You ask him to wait a minute. Doesn't he want to look at your x-rays? Your medical record?

"No," he replies, "I trust Fassnacht [your doctor] implicitly. If she says you need surgery, I'm ready to do it." You say that replacing a knee sounds like an awfully drastic step. What's involved?

"We just cut the old knee out and put the new one in." You ask if you will be able to walk, to climb stairs, to ride your bike as you used to like to do.

"Sure. I'll make sure that you'll have no limitations." You are worried by the surgeon's offhand manner and tell him that you want a second opinion. He scowls. "My schedule fills up pretty fast, and that knee is deteriorating further every second. I might not be able to get you in when you absolutely have to have it." You stand firm and tell him that you will call him when you get a second opinion. You make some calls and get the names of doctors who give second opinions. One of them is Vanessa Virtuevessel, M.D., an orthopedic surgeon in a group practice with three other surgeons at a local clinic. You call for a second opinion appointment. The nurse tells you that she will mail you a form to sign so that Fassnacht can release your records and x-rays. When you go to the clinic, you discover that Virtuevessel has your chart spread out on her desk and x-rays up on the light box. Even you can see that the knee doesn't look good. As she examines you, you explain that you were uncomfortable with the surgeon's breezy approach and too-deft answers.

Virtuevessel says, "I'm sorry that Dr. Kowboi made you feel uneasy. He's a bit like that sometimes. We surgeons sometimes cut first and ask questions later. But I think both Dr. Fassnacht and Dr. Kowboi are right. You've had reasonable trials of all the drugs you can tolerate. Your rheumatoid factor—a measure of how severe the disease is—is quite high. I think we ought to replace the knee."

You are immediately calmed by Virtuevessel's manner. You ask if she can do the surgery. She replies that as the source of the second opinion, she can't ethically do it. You ask her to recommend someone else. She tells you that any of the other two orthopedic surgeons in the group can handle knee replacements.

"You should understand," she adds, "that we're a partnership, and I will receive some of the surgery fee in the form of profits at the end of the year. We also rent space to a physical therapist. If you use him, I will receive some of the rent. If this makes you uncomfortable, I can recommend someone outside our group." You're impressed with her honesty and tell her that someone from the group will be fine—if they're good.

"Both of them are board-certified. We have their resumes on file with the nurse, if you want to see them." You ask if there are any statistics on their results. Virtuevessel makes a face. "The state just made us start keeping numbers on that. The nurse has the file." You ask about the usefulness of the new knee. Virtuevessel says that with good healing, you will eventually be able to walk and climb stairs and ride the bike, but you will have to set the seat high to avoid too much bending of the artificial knee.

You look at the statistics on her two partners. You notice that even though both have good results, Norman Noscrub, M.D., has had many more patients with postoperative infections than the other, Stanley Sterildrape, M.D. You decide on Sterildrape.

You ask Fassnacht to be in charge of your overall care in the hospital. You have filed a **living will** and want to make sure that your wishes are carried out if anything goes wrong. Since Fassnacht has agreed to your wishes, you want her in control of the team of doctors treating you. The hospital records her as the "physician in charge" of your case. Everything goes well, and after a few months of rehabilitation, you are back on the bike.

This is an idealized picture to some degree, but it represents what *should* happen when the patient and the patient's chosen doctor are in control and nothing happens without their approval. If you don't feel that your situation meets these criteria, do not allow the doctor to pass go. Negotiate and, if you can't win, seek another doctor.

The Doctor's Criteria for Success and Failure (and Yours)

This may seem to be a strange subject to raise. Don't doctors know when a treatment has succeeded or failed? Generally, yes. Aren't the criteria—what to look for—to determine success or failure set by the medical profession? Not at all.

We've all seen at least one television movie in which the life (or appearance or sanity) of a patient was saved because one doctor kept on pushing after all his colleagues had given up. There is much truth in this fiction. Doctors are people, and they differ. Some of them will try any new thing that they read about in the medical journal that arrived yesterday afternoon. Others will not adopt new treatments until they feel that the treatment is completely proven and most other doctors have adopted them.

Some pore over the medical journals like pirates in search of buried treasure. Others have read nothing in years, choose their continuing education courses by the quality of the resort at which they are held and sleep through the classes. Some prescribe with abandon, believing that "there's a pill for everything." Others are so afraid of the negative side effects of drugs in the elderly that they neglect drugs that could be useful. Some surgeons think internists are unduly cerebral and cautious to a fault. Some internists think surgeons live by the motto "If it moves, cut it." One cardiologist may prescribe smoking cessation, weight loss, a walking program and nitroglycerin tablets. Another may prescribe the same, plus a triple bypass.

Some strive to treat the whole person and are satisfied with a patient who has avoided the risks of surgery and is handling his condition well on medical therapy. Others see no irony in the claim that "the operation was a success, but the patient died."

This wide variety of approaches is not necessarily bad (it gives you the option of shopping around), and it does not mean that doctors know nothing. It simply indicates that medicine is, as Lewis Thomas, M.D., wrote, "the youngest science." Various experts have estimated that it was not until somewhere between 1920 and 1950 that one had an equal chance of being helped or harmed by an encounter with a doctor. Before that, one was more likely to be harmed.

Medicine has also evolved (some would disagree about the choice of verb) into a bewildering variety of specialties and subspecialties. Most assume that if a patient has been referred to them (or has called for an appointment), choosing them was obviously the right thing to do, and they will plow ahead until it becomes obvious that they are not helping. "If you go to Midas, you get a muffler," is the way one doctor has put it.

Doctors respond to peer pressure (as do all people) and tend to practice like their colleagues practice. The gang at the hospital across town may have a completely different approach.

The upshot is that you have to find out what it is the doctor is trying to do for you and tell him whether that is what you want. We can't stress one point strongly enough: Nothing in a doctor's training equips him to make the choice for you. Nothing in his training makes him better able to make the choice than you can. Doctors don't share their standards of success and failure with patients because they have never realized that you have your own standards. They are parents; you are a child. The prejudices we described above get in the way, too.

It's up to you to find out two things:

- What outcome does the doctor expect and accept?

- What are the alternatives?

A patient may feel that what the doctor has recommended—say, medical treatment and use of a portable oxygen tank—is a fine outcome and preferable to the 20 percent risk of death and the 15 percent risk of a worsened condition attached to surgery. But the doctor may well have recommended this because success, for him, is keeping the patient out of the operating room. Another patient may decide that anything is preferable to being attached to an oxygen tank for the rest of his life and will accept the doctor's recommendation for surgery. The *doctor* may have recommended this because, for him, success is avoiding dependence on oxygen. The reasons the doctor recommends a treatment may have nothing to do with the way *you* look at it.

People tend to think that because a doctor recommends something, he must know how to balance medical considerations with considerations of the "quality of life" based on some more or less objective set of values shared with the patient. Nothing could be further from the truth.

A doctor's education is usually exclusively in medicine or the sciences that make up the foundation for medicine unless his undergraduate professors or the medical school has decided to help him be a more broadly educated human being somewhere along the line. The doctor may have no acquaintance with the humanities, philosophy, values, literature, art, music or history. The typical doctor is probably less well equipped to deal with issues of value and choice than the typical English major. The upshot: Find out what your doctor is thinking and why—then make your own choices.

How Sure of the Diagnosis Is the Doctor? How Did He Get to It?

Some diagnoses are obvious; many are not. The diagnosis recorded at hospital admission is wrong about 40 percent of the time.[1] A portion of this admission diagnosis error rate reflects the current state of medicine and not necessarily a failing on the part of the doctor. (Even the suspicion of some diagnoses such as a heart attack or a ruptured appendix is a good reason to send someone to the hospital; tests done in the hospital may establish some other diagnosis as correct, but the decision to hospitalize, based on the knowledge the doctor had at the time, was correct.) Another portion is simply error, sometimes fatal error.

Is Overtesting or Undertesting the Problem?

Autopsy results show that there is always a certain percentage of cases in which a diagnosis of an incurable, fatal disease is made when the correct diagnosis is a disease that is not fatal if treated. Since the diagnosis led to no treatment or only palliative treatment, the patients in these cases died unnecessarily. The few studies that have been done on this issue show that *the percentage of these types of cases has probably been rising over the last three decades*. It reached 10 percent of cases in a study done in the early 1980s. To put it in the most forceful terms possible: Misdiagnosis accounts for 10 percent of all deaths in which the patient died in the hospital. At least as measured by this kind of fatal mistake, the problem of misdiagnosis is getting worse, not better.[2]

---

[1] Alan Brewster, M.D., personal oral communication. Other studies have shown diagnosis error rates of 10 percent to 81 percent, depending on study methods. See, for example, the studies cited by Charles B. Inlander, Lowell Levin and Ed Weiner in *Medicine on Trial* (New York: Prentice-Hall, 1988), pp. 67-80.

[2] H. H. R. Friederici and M. Sebastian, *Archives of Pathology Laboratory Medicine,* (June 1984): 521, cited in Inlander et al., *Medicine on Trial,* p. 72.

What can you do to protect yourself and ensure that you get the best (and right) treatment? You need to get your doctor to share her diagnostic thinking with you. What else did she think you might have? What is in favor of the diagnosis she chose? How sure is she? What test results—if any—tipped the scales in favor of one diagnosis over another? How does the diagnosis affect the treatment? What else can she do to make the diagnosis more certain?

You can help deal with the problem of misdiagnosis by keeping several points in mind: First, symptoms may be real and troubling to you, but they do not necessarily indicate something that can, or should, be medically treated. The labor that accompanies the birth of a child is painful, but pregnancy is not a disease. Many people have a tendency to somatize—to express problems in their lives as physical symptoms. The symptom can be reduced by drugs, but it will not go away until the problem is solved. An understanding friend may be better equipped to help than a doctor. Sometimes even talking to a pet may be of more value than everything in the pharmacy. It's ultimately up to each individual to know the difference. The doctor can only help by communicating what the tests show.

The second point is this: Doctors talk about the "sensitivity" and the "specificity" of tests. Sensitivity refers to the ability of the test to detect *something,* regardless of what it is. Specificity refers to how accurately the test distinguishes between the various somethings that might be there. The ideal test is 100 percent sensitive—it detects something every time something is present—and is specific to only one something. Every test in existence falls short of this ideal. Many, in addition to being less than 100 percent sensitive—that is, they miss something that is really there—give "false positives," indicating that something is wrong when it isn't. Most are less than specific—they narrow the possibilities to a few things, assuming something is really there, but they don't tell which one. For example, elevated amounts of enzymes produced by the liver can indicate that a person has liver damage or that he is taking one of the many drugs that harmlessly elevate the level of these enzymes.

Since perfect tests don't exist, doctors have to use the ones they have. Almost all tests have some risk associated with them. So the dilemma arises: "For $200 worth of tests, and a small amount of risk, I am 97 percent sure of what this patient has. For $2,000 more, and more risk, I can be 99 percent sure. Is it worth it?"

Worth it for whom? You? The doctor? Her malpractice insurer? Many doctors say that they do more testing than they feel is wise simply to protect themselves from malpractice suits. Taken at face value, this means that *doctors think they are doing too many tests now. If they considered only their patients' welfare, they would do fewer.*

This suggests that the problem you face, as a patient, is not under-testing that may miss a diagnosis—even though the results from the autopsy studies we mentioned are disturbing. The danger you face is *overtesting*. Pennsylvania Blue Cross and Blue Shield apparently agree; they have decided to pay for some tests only in special situations.

What can you do to protect yourself?

- At each step of the process, ask your doctor why she is doing each test and what information she expects to gain from it.

- Ask her about the risks associated with it.

- Ask her how sure she is of the diagnosis now, and ask her to express it in percentage terms. If she says she is more than 50 percent sure, ask how sure she expects to be as a result of the test. If she indicates less than 85 percent certainty, ask how the test will narrow the diagnostic range.

- Most important, ask her why she can't make the diagnosis from your history alone.

Don't let her proceed until you're satisfied.

Surgery and the Medical Alternatives; Medicine and the Surgical Alternatives

Surgery is serious business. But so is medicine. Researchers Paul Gertman and Knight Steele did a study of **iatrogenesis**—doctor-induced illness—on a medical service (a division of a hospital that primarily offers one branch of medicine such as internal medicine, cardiac care or surgery) at Boston University Hospital. They found that more than one-third of the patients had some doctor-caused illness, the severity ranging from mild to fatal. Nine percent had doctor-caused illnesses that were either disfiguring or life threatening. Two percent died. Gertman and Steele used very strict criteria for iatrogenesis and noted that their results probably underestimated the actual occurrence.

So medical treatment and surgery are both risky. Avoiding the danger is not a simple matter of staying out of the operating room. In negotiating the risks and benefits of both surgery and medical treatment, you need to figure out your doctor's reasoning, just as you had to do with the matter of diagnosis. Again, there are no right and wrong answers here that the doctor learned in medical school. Balancing the risks and benefits is ultimately your decision.

First, you need to find out what your doctor thinks a good outcome is. You may be surprised at how little improvement she will be satisfied with. (Example: Parkinson's disease, a disorder in which uncontrollable trembling and twitching of the hands and loss of coordination develops, is primarily a disease of those over 60. It can often be controlled with drugs, but these have significant side effects. With constant monitoring and surgical therapy [if necessary], most patients can achieve a high degree of control of symptoms. But they won't if the doctor considers reduction of hand tremors as the best possible outcome and does not work at balancing the drugs used or consider surgery.)

After you've squared expectations with the doctor, you need to find out how beneficial, and how risky, the various medical and surgical alternatives are likely to be. This is your decision, not the doctor's. His job is to give you the facts. Even so, it's important to recognize that overall, surgery is generally riskier than medical treatment. There is another virtue to the conservative approach that many internists take: It is usually, although not always, possible to proceed with surgery after a trial of medical therapy. The reverse may not be possible—the offending organ may have been removed.

You should understand the one big exception to this advice is cancer. For some tumors, medical therapy may be the best approach, but, in general, it is best to surgically remove suspected malignancies as soon as possible. The primary reason is that cancers can metastasize, or spread, throughout the body. Cancers that have metastasized are much harder to treat. The secondary reason is that tumors grow, and what can be a minor operation that leaves an inconspicuous scar for a small tumor may turn into a major, disfiguring surgery if it is allowed to grow. Even in these cases, the approaches taken by various experts may differ. You need to know the risks and benefits of each.

Let's say that you need surgery. The first thing you should do is find out all you can about the type of operation that will probably be used in your case.

The second thing you should do is obtain a second opinion for nonurgent, or elective, procedures. You should get this second opinion from someone other than the surgeon who will do the surgery and who is not connected financially with the doctor who recommended it. This is something you should ask about, even though the second-opinion doctor should disclose any financial connection he has with the one who recommended surgery. You should obtain from the second physician the same sort of information you received (or tried to get) from the first: risks and benefits of the various courses of treatment.

You should seek a third opinion if the second opinion does not concur with the first. Find out why there is disagreement. Most often there will be lack of consensus because the medical profession hasn't agreed on a right (or wrong) approach. But there may be doubt about the diagnosis. (For example, an internist feels a lump in your breast and suggests that you see a surgeon for a needle biopsy, an in-office procedure in which a fine, hollow needle is used to remove a tiny bit of tissue for examination. The surgeon can't feel the lump and suggests that you have a mammogram. The mammogram, as is usually the case with older women, shows all sorts of changes, none of them particularly benign and none of them clearly suggestive of cancer. The surgeon refers you back to the internist, who can feel no lump this time. Nothing has been established, you're worried, and both doctors are concerned and embarrassed. A third opinion, perhaps from an oncologist [a specialist in the treatment of cancer], could help.)

Suppose you decide on surgery. The job is still not finished. You should insist on seeing the **anesthesiologist** or **anesthetist** who will give the anesthesia. You should ask what he will do if the first approach, for some reason, does not work. (For example, the anesthetist decides on spinal anesthesia but can't get the needle into the spinal canal, so he uses a general anesthetic instead.)

You should ask about preoperative sedation (a shot or pill to relax you before you go to surgery) and plans for repeating it if you do not get to the operating room on time. (For example, you are scheduled for removal of a portion of an enlarged prostate gland via a cystoscope [a hollow tube that can be inserted into the bladder through the penis, and through which an instrument can be used to remove diseased prostate and bladder tissue]. You have been very worried about this ever since the urologist [a surgeon specializing in operations on the kidneys, bladder and urinary tract] described the procedure to you. You're told that you will be heavily sedated for this and possibly out completely if you respond to the drug that way. You're given a shot, after which you spend a pleasant, dreamy hour lying on the gurney. An emergency case bollixes the operating room schedule, and you are taken in two hours late—more awake than you've ever been in your life.) The anesthesiologist or anesthetist will usually be happy to write an order for repeating the preoperative sedation if you remind him.

You should, of course, make him aware of any drug allergies that you may have. Sometimes an allergy to one drug means potential problems with a whole class of drugs.

The preoperative consent form that you will be asked to sign may have a clause in it allowing the surgeon to perform any procedure he deems necessary after he gets "inside." Signing such a broad operative consent completely defeats all the careful effort that you have devoted to making sure that you stay in control of your treatment. Your surgeon has a pretty good idea of what he will find when he starts; if you discuss limiting the operative consent to those things *when you agree to surgery* (not when the consent form is handed to you in the hospital), he may be willing to eliminate the overly broad clause.

To sum up:

- Make sure you know what outcome from the surgery is expected and what can go wrong.

- Ask for the possible results in numerical terms—85 percent chance of a good result, 15 percent chance of a bad one and the like. Don't accept general reassurances like "everything will be fine."

- Don't sign a blanket operative consent.

- Insist on seeing the anesthesiologist. Let him know about allergies, make arrangements for repeating preoperative sedation, and make sure you understand what arrangements have been made for alternative anesthesia.

Specialists

Today more doctors are specialists than generalists. The all-purpose doctor of yore is today a minority. There are at least two reasons for this: First, the specialties are far more lucrative than internal medicine, general practice and family practice. Second, because the general fields are so broad, and an internist's training in particular overlaps those of other specialties, residencies in these fields are very demanding. (A residency is a period of time, usually three to five years, spent in training at a hospital before a doctor obtains certification from one of the numerous national medical boards that she is adequately trained in her field.) Also demanding is practice, once the doctor is into it. The fact is that a doctor has much more control over her time if she is an eye surgeon, limited to one type of treatment for one organ, than if she is an internist, whose purview is any nonsurgical treatment of anything.

As we noted earlier, the fee-for-service system is heavily biased in favor of procedures, discrete and well-defined things that a doctor can do, usually of a surgical nature. Cognitive skills such as making the diagnosis that may avoid an unnecessary operation costing tens of thousands are far less well rewarded. So the United States has too many surgeons and not enough generalists. The medical students go where the livin' is easiest.

You face different situations when you are referred to a specialist as an outpatient and when you are hospitalized.

Outpatient Referrals: Some abuses of referrals have taken place under Medicare (and other insurance systems). The most common is called "Ping-Ponging," when a specialist and a generalist refer a patient back and forth between them, getting a fee at each visit, while the patient flies across town like a Ping-Pong ball across the table. Generally, referrals to specialists should be for a limited term and should only be done for specialized diagnostic testing, treatment or consultation requested by a primary care physician.

You can save yourself needless repeat testing, exposure to multiple x-rays and the like if you make sure that a copy of your medical record and test results (including x-ray films) is either mailed to the specialist in advance or given to you to take with you to the appointment. This is simple common sense, but it rarely happens. The specialist may have no more to go on than what was said in the initial phone call from your doctor. Insist that your records and test results get to the specialist no later than you do.

The simple answer is for you to obtain a *current* copy of your medical record. This is yet another case in which patients have to do something the doctors *should* be doing in order to make sure it gets done at all. You have a definite right to your medical record in only a few states, and even then there are restrictions. We suggest that you find a consumer-oriented doctor who will request the records and then give you a copy. It's the simplest, cheapest and fastest way.

If you are referred more than once to the same specialist, or to another specialist for what seems to be the same reason, stop your doctor and ask why the referrals are going on. Don't accept another one unless you are satisfied with the reasons. If your doctor is referring you because she genuinely does not feel competent to perform the service the specialist is providing, fine; a doctor who knows her limits is a wonderful thing. But if these are not the reasons, each referral is costing you unnecessarily, even if all the doctors involved take assignment. Again, you should be the judge and decide for yourself whether to see the specialist to whom you're referred.

Specialists in the Hospital: Your situation in the hospital is different. There are services and departments within hospitals such as medicine, surgery, intensive care, trauma, geriatrics and so on. Let's say that your doctor admits you for medical treatment of a problem. You are admitted under her care to the general medical service, the part of the hospital that handles general problems that don't fall under some specialty such as obstetrics or psychiatry. If it is a teaching hospital, a corps of residents, senior medical students and nurses-in-training will descend upon you. Many of them will be charged with some aspect of your care and will be reading your chart to carry out orders or writing more orders in your chart for others to carry out. If you don't have a personal physician in the area and have been admitted under the care of the house staff, you are fair game for all of the residents and all of the attending physicians on the service.

Additional testing reveals that you need surgery. You are transferred to the surgical service. Let's say that you have medical problems that are complicated enough to require continuing care by an internist, even as preparations for surgery go on. You will now have the residents and senior students of the surgical service on the case as well. An attending physician who is called in as a consultant and becomes interested in your case ("good teaching material") will stay on it and bill for the visits that satisfy her curiosity unless she is told to stay away by whoever's in charge (who may be hard to identify). The medical myth working here is that since every doctor works to the highest standard and the hospital oversees them all, you are safe even if no one is obviously in charge.

Some hospitals have recognized that the situation we have described is fraught with risk. They are designating a "physician in charge" of each case who is supposed to coordinate everything done by everybody. If you, or someone who has your power of attorney (a legal document giving him the power to act for you in certain situations) in the event you are too ill to exercise control, are not in charge, *no one* may be.

Another reason one person should be in charge is to make sure that all of your doctors accept assignment; otherwise, you could find yourself responsible for additional out-of-pocket expenses up to the balance billing limit. In the earlier example on page 115, you avoided an additional $265 out-of-pocket expense when the doctor accepted assignment and did not charge you the balance billing limit.

Without an advocate to negotiate assignment with your doctors, you could be responsible for thousands of dollars in additional out-of-pocket expenses.

Advance Directives

Death and dying have always been major human preoccupations; many psychologists have noted that people (at least in developed Western countries in the late twentieth century) spend the first half of their lives trying to deal with their adolescence and the last half trying to come to terms with death.

One of the more dubious achievements of late-twentieth-century medicine has been the development of the ability to delay death almost inevitably. It can be delayed long after a person has entered a permanent vegetative state and will never exercise any of the faculties that make him human again. Even after the brain stem has lost the ability to control breathing, even after the heart has lost the ability to beat on its own, "life" of a sort can be continued with respirators and pacemakers. The artificial heart, which may someday be used to keep potential organ donors "alive" indefinitely, can be called in if these fail. Some people resist all the technology and die anyway; one cynical physician has expressed it as "You die, but you die with your electrolytes in balance."

Doctors, who are often so ready to inject their value judgments into treatment decisions with no formal training to do so, have shrunk from it here. They have forced most decisions in this area into the courts, and the case law that is developing is quite clear: You *always* have a right to refuse treatment—of any sort—if you are mentally competent and have not fallen into the clutches of a hospital. This principle, at least, is well established: The competent individual can refuse to *begin* treatment. The cases that have garnered so much attention recently have been about stopping treatments already begun.

The evolving case law suggests that even "treatments" such as supplying food or water, which one or more of your doctors may regard as merely humane measures designed to comfort you, are not part of medical practice per se. If you are not mentally competent, the recent cases suggest, the wishes you expressed while competent must be respected. (Of course, expressing those wishes in a formal way via a living will or **durable power of attorney** can avoid a host of problems. For more information, obtain a copy of *Medicare Advance Directives,* [HCFA publication 02175], available at any Social Security office.)

Quality of Life: Is It Worth the Living?

Deciding how you want to be treated at the end of your life requires some imagination and rather fearless self-analysis. First, recognize that experience of illness and the medical world, for most people, is rather limited. One should not judge one's ability to accept pain on the basis of a visit to the dentist, with novocaine and nitrous oxide. Pain has heights that most people will never scale. (Ask anyone who has passed a kidney stone.) Relief for pain is limited to what the doctor feels he can prescribe without killing you. Whatever that dose is, the nurses will give less because they are afraid of addiction, even if you have two weeks to live. An *extremely* painful condition is unlikely to be given adequate relief in a hospital. (A hospice is another matter. See chapter 7.)

Even if you are not in real pain, you may be acutely uncomfortable. A nasogastric tube that moves constantly and irritates the throat with each swallow; a dry mouth and cracked lips that result from being denied any more fluid than ice chips; a catheter that creates the sensation of having to urinate desperately, even while it drains urine; and intravenous lines that prevent you from using your hands or bending your arms plus the sensation of whatever incision you've had, even if there's no pain until you move, are triple-distilled misery. Add the pain of cancer and nausea from chemotherapy to the mix, and one has a "quality of life" that many would argue is not worth living unless there is the hope of a cure.

Your Rights Right Now

A 28-year-old quadriplegic woman suffering from severe cerebral palsy and arthritis sufficiently painful to require morphine, Elizabeth Bouvia, was in almost this same situation (substitute the pain of severe arthritis for the cancer), and she petitioned a California court to let her die. She was being kept alive by feedings through a nasogastric tube. She asked to have the tube removed, which would eventually lead to death by starvation. The hospital and her doctors refused. The California Second Circuit Court of Appeals ruled that, as an article in the *New England Journal of Medicine* paraphrased it, "a patient need not be comatose or terminally ill to refuse medical treatment, even when the treatment may be lifesaving and even when its absence may lead to an earlier death. The court added that the right to refuse medical treatment was virtually absolute and the patient's motives were not a matter for debate or decision by others."

The *Bouvia* case is important because it is the only one to date in which a conscious, coherent individual requested the withdrawal of medical treatment solely on quality-of-life grounds and was upheld in court. Other cases having to do with artificial feeding and hydration are important because they are rapidly establishing a judicial and medical consensus that, as the same article put it:

*The focus of discussion should be the patient's wishes, not the type of treatment or the patient's prognosis. Artificial feeding can be viewed on a level with other medical interventions—cardiopulmonary resuscitation (CPR), mechanical ventilation, dialysis and antibiotic therapy. It should not be considered a part of "ordinary care" or the routine provision of nursing care and comfort. Competent patients have the right to refuse this treatment after assessing for themselves the benefits and burdens. This right is not limited to comatose or terminally ill patients. For incompetent patients, feeding, like other treatments, can be stopped in accordance with the patient's previously expressed wishes. (*New England Journal of Medicine *318 [1988]: 288)*

This consensus is, however, an *emerging* one, not firmly fixed in law, and will probably be subject to much attempted cutting and trimming. For the moment, however, what these cases establish—after much needless suffering and expense on the part of the persons and families involved—is that courts in several states are inclined to view patients' own assessments of their quality of life as the deciding factor in refusing or stopping treatment. The Supreme Court's refusal to review one of these cases, *Brophy v. New England Sinai Hospital,* indicates that it would be inclined to agree. The *New England Journal of Medicine* paraphrased the court's decision this way:

*The state had no duty to preserve life when the patient would feel that the means of doing so demeaned his or her humanity. Only Brophy could make decisions about the quality of his life—not physicians or third parties, including the court. . . . Even though he was not terminally ill, he had the right to refuse life-sustaining treatments, including artificial feeding. . . . The discontinuation of Brophy's feeding would not represent suicide or direct killing, the court ruled, nor would it subject him to a painful death by starvation. Instead, it would merely allow the underlying disease to take its natural course. (*New England Journal of Medicine *318 [1988]: 287)*

Again, what applies to artificial feeding applies even more strongly to respirators and artificial hearts. You have a constitutional right to refuse any medical treatment.

Having the right does not mean that others will honor it. It is probably safe to assume that in the current state of the law, you or your family will have to bear at least some legal expenses and needless anguish if you do not take definite steps to make sure that your doctor knows your wishes and is willing to honor them.

Thanks to organizations such as Choice in Dying, every state now has legislation recognizing **advance directives** (living wills and durable powers of attorney for health care). These documents allow people to prepare for their future health care if they become unable to make their own medical decisions. We suggest that you contact Choice in Dying at 800-989-WILL to obtain an advance directives packet that complies with your state's law.

Given the current state of the law, we believe that you should both establish a living will and execute a durable power of attorney, giving control of decisions about your health care to a trusted friend or relative in the event you are no longer able to make them. The living will allows you to specify exactly what you mean, and doing both covers all bases. Phrases such as "no heroic measures" and "no artificial life support" are too vague to be enforceable on your doctors and the hospital and will in all likelihood land the matter back in court, which is what you want to avoid.

There is one area in which you, the doctor and the hospital will wind up speaking the same language without much effort: "no-code" orders. This means "Do no attempt cardiopulmonary resuscitation"—if your heart stops, let it stay stopped. You can specify to your doctor that you do or do not want a no-code order written. Perhaps the most relevant (and well-hidden) fact here is that only about 4 percent of patients who have cardiopulmonary resuscitation are discharged from the hospital alive. In that sense, contrary to what we see on television, it's a procedure that has a 96 percent failure rate.

In this chapter you will learn: How review agencies can get you into, or keep you out of, the hospital ▪ How to contact the peer review organization in your area ▪ How to make an ally of your doctor ▪ How to request reconsideration and appeals ▪ When to file a request for an expedited review ▪ How to request a hearing before an administrative law judge

6. Medicare and Hospitals

The purpose of this chapter is to explain how to make sure you get what you are entitled to under Medicare from hospitals. Chapter 2 explained the Diagnosis-Related Groups (DRG) system, which is the way Medicare currently makes payments to hospitals. Chapter 5 explained how to negotiate with your doctor and the hospital about your treatment. This chapter is a legalistic one, designed to show you how to make sure Medicare pays for the care you need.

Review Organizations and Your Care

There is a lot of variation among regions of the country in the rate at which people of all ages are admitted to hospitals and in what they are admitted for. Research has shown that this has little to do with the demographics of the populations being served—with how old people are, how sick they are and so on. It has much more to do with the practice patterns of the doctors in a community. It is also affected to some extent by the availability of hospital beds. For this and other related reasons, Medicare and other insurers are working hard to discourage unnecessary hospitalization. They are also concerned with getting people out as soon as they are ready to go, either home or to a skilled nursing facility.

The mechanisms that Medicare uses to deal with this problem have evolved over the years, the Joint Commission on Accreditation of Healthcare Organizations has added others, and the DRG system brought the peer review organizations (PROs) with it. These are layered on top of one another. For the first time in Medicare's history, the PROs are involved in deciding whether or not you can get into the hospital as well as when you have to leave. And, of course, your doctor has a lot to do with whether or not you go into the hospital. We discuss the roles of each of these in turn.

Your Doctor

The medical profession is losing its control over American health care. Experts differ over whether this is a good or bad thing and about the extent of the loss. Most agree that it has happened because the medical profession is seen by many opinion leaders as having broken the "social contract" that gave it that control in exchange for selfless dedication to people's health. At the same time, technology has made it possible to render in the doctor's office or in an ambulatory surgery center much care that formerly could be given only in a hospital. This has meant that there are new income opportunities for doctors. For example, they can operate on you in an ambulatory surgery center in which they have part ownership and receive fees for the use of the facilities that formerly would have gone to the hospital. Your doctor is being pulled in many different directions.

Generally, a doctor who wants to keep you out of the hospital is a good thing. What is important for you is that you understand what your options are and why the doctor is proposing to treat you outside the hospital.

The most important thing to discuss is any reason why you think you should be treated in the hospital; make sure you understand the doctor's reasons and agree with them. You are always free to seek another doctor, even in a managed care plan such as a Medicare+Choice plan.

In some cases the PRO decides that a patient's surgery must be performed outside the hospital. We tell you what to do about that a little later.

The Hospital Utilization Review Committee

One of the requirements for hospitals to be accredited is to have a committee of doctors that looks at utilization of services, generically called utilization review committees, or URCs. (Some hospitals give them slightly different names.) The PRO can elect to delegate some or all of its review responsibilities for individual cases to the URC of a hospital if it believes that the URC is performing well. So you may get a notice regarding your care, before or after you enter the hospital, from the URC, from the PRO or from the URC-acting-as-PRO. (The stationery the notice is on will be different.)

Medicare+Choice Plans

Medicare+Choice plans operate in the same way as other review organizations; they make determinations regarding the benefits a Medicare enrollee receives. They are also required by law to advise enrollees of their right to appeal any decision relating to treatment or the denial of care. In a Medicare+Choice plan, the initial level of review is the plan itself rather than the PRO, intermediary or carrier.

Beneficiaries who are dissatisfied with the initial determination made by their Medicare+Choice plans have the right to request a **reconsideration**. The request for reconsideration is the first step in the appeals process. Medicare regulations require Medicare+Choice plans to conduct both standard and expedited reconsiderations.

Your Employee or Retiree Health Plan

Several years ago Congress made Medicare the *secondary* payer for Medicare beneficiaries who are still working and have health insurance through their employer or who are retired and continue to receive comprehensive health insurance from their employer. This change made employers sit up and take notice of retiree health costs. Many have established preadmission and postadmission review procedures or hired firms to review the cost and quality of care they pay for. These may affect your hospital stay.

Peer Review Organizations

Medicare's continuing attempt to control the costs and monitor the quality of health care for Medicare beneficiaries is the PROs. PROs are groups of doctors who have contracts with Medicare to review various aspects of treatment Medicare pays for. Usually one PRO covers an entire state or a large portion of it. The idea is that the medical profession will remain self-policing because the reviewers are doctors; at the same time, Medicare can obligate them to focus on what it considers to be problem areas through contracts. The PROs are supposed to work toward targets—for example: "Unnecessary hospital admissions should be reduced by 35 percent over the next two years." The key term for Medicare is "35 percent"; the key word for the doctors is "unnecessary."

How the two perspectives work together determines what the PRO in a particular area is concentrating on at any given time. The areas currently under review around the nation include the following:

- Reviews of proposed hospital admissions for various procedures

- Reviews of lengthy hospital or skilled nursing facility stays

- Reviews of discharges, readmissions and deaths

- Reviews of charts after discharge, to measure the appropriateness of admissions and the quality of care given

Medicare Intermediaries and Carriers

Medicare's intermediaries and carriers have review responsibilities, too, basically related to oddities that show up during their processing of claims. These functions overlap those of the PROs and the URCs to some extent.

The First Hurdle: Getting In

The following review bodies could make decisions regarding your hospitalization:

- Your doctor

- The hospital's utilization review committee

- Medicare+Choice plans

- Your employee or retiree health plan reviewer

- The peer review organization

- Intermediaries and carriers

In reading the rest of this section, it is important to remember that *only your doctor, the hospital utilization review committee or your Medicare+Choice plan, acting in accordance with medical staff bylaws, can deny your admission to the hospital.* Even if your employee or retiree health plan denies you admission, there's a good chance that Medicare will cover the service (for this reason, we strongly advise that you sign up for Medicare Parts A and B when you are eligible). The PRO can review your request only if you have been denied admission by your doctor, the hospital or your Medicare+Choice plan and you decide to appeal the decision. The intermediaries and carriers decide whether they will pay for the hospital stay or the services provided. *You are always free to seek admission to the hospital if you think you need it.*

Your Doctor

If your doctor decides that you do not need hospital care, you can discuss it with him or find another doctor. There are no avenues of appeal that result in someone giving your doctor an order to admit you against his will. You probably would not want to be treated by a doctor who is being forced to do something against his better judgment anyway. You can, of course, ask for a second opinion, and the doctor rendering it may be able to convince your doctor that you do need hospitalization.

The Hospital's Utilization Review Committee

It is unlikely, but not impossible, that you will be informed that your admission to the hospital will not be accepted by the hospital's URC. There are really only two instances: In the first the PRO has delegated review of proposed admissions and procedures to the hospital's URC. In the second the URC will be reviewing your doctor's cases for admission because of some problems he has had with unnecessary admissions in the past or—more rarely still—if the hospital's URC is reviewing all nonemergency admissions because of problems in the past or a PRO mandate. Hospitals are so hungry for bed-filling patients now that any hospital-initiated preadmission review is unlikely.

Two different situations need to be carefully distinguished here: If the hospital's URC is acting on its own, you have no appeal without your doctor's help. Your doctor's right to admit you is limited by the hospital's bylaws and the conditions of his membership in the medical staff. Generally, these do not allow him to admit cases the URC says should not be admitted.

If the URC is acting as the agent of the PRO, things are different. *You have a right to appeal the PRO's decision.* We cover how in an upcoming section on PROs.

Medicare+Choice Plans

Medicare+Choice plans are responsible for determining the appropriateness of all the medical services you receive, and this includes hospital inpatient services. Accordingly, they review treatment decisions made by your physician and may, under certain circumstances, deny you admission to the hospital.

As with all review bodies, you have the right to a **standard review** of your plan's decisions concerning your care.

Your Employee or Retiree Health Plan Reviewer

If your employee or retiree health plan reviewer decides that the plan will not pay for hospital care, Medicare still pays for what the employer plan does not cover as long as the services you need are Medicare-covered and medically necessary. *The employee or retiree health plan review has no effect on Medicare's decisions.* If this situation arises, we suggest that you contact your employer and your doctor. Your employee or retiree health plan will have some procedure for appeals, and you should pursue this channel first if your situation is not an emergency. The first rejection may have come from a computer, a nurse reviewer, a doctor or a combination of all three. In cases that are appealed, most of the review entities make use of expert physician consultants to decide cases in order to protect themselves from liability. A rejection of an appeal from one of these services generally is solid evidence that you do not need hospitalization. You should ask your doctor about the medical necessity for the treatment he proposes.

If your appeal is denied, you or your doctor should contact the Medicare intermediary or carrier and ask if there is a problem with the admission since your (current or former) employer refused to pay. Generally, you will be told that Medicare will cover the treatment and that the carrier and your employer will fight it out later. This is a tricky area that is not exactly the responsibility of any one of Medicare's review agents right now. You should document all your contacts with your employer and the reviewer in writing. A suggested appeal letter is shown below.

Sample Appeal Letter for Rejection of Admission Request by an Employee or Retiree Health Plan Reviewer

Your name
Your street address
Your city, state and ZIP code

Date *(Important!)*

Office to which appeals are addressed
Street address
City, state and ZIP code
ATTN: Proper person, if any

REFERENCE: Your employer/retiree medical plan number
               Your Medicare number

Dear Madam or Sir:

   I have been advised that you have rejected my doctor's plans to hospitalize me for *[name of condition or operation or both]*.

My physician, Dr. _____ , feels strongly that I should be treated in the fashion he has suggested. I am attaching a letter from him, plus additional medical evidence (if any) in support of my request for a reconsideration of your decision.

I look forward to hearing from you.

Sincerely yours,
Your signature

Your doctor will usually handle such appeals for you, but you can strengthen the case for review and add pressure to the reviewers by acting on your own.

The Peer Review Organization

As explained earlier, the PROs have been set up to measure, preserve and, one hopes, improve the quality of care under Medicare. They can do anything within their contracts in this field that the Medicare law permits. The law permits them to deny you admission under the following circumstances:

- There is a problem with unnecessary admissions in your area, and Medicare has contracted with the PRO for a preadmission review service.

- You are scheduled to have one of the procedures for which second opinions, preadmission review or outpatient surgery is required, and one or more conditions have not been met.

If you are denied admission by a PRO preadmission review or by a decision that your operation must be done in an outpatient facility, you can request a reconsideration. The instructions at the end of this chapter explain how.

Intermediaries and Carriers

Intermediaries and carriers are insurance companies that have contracts with Medicare to process Part A and Part B claims. Intermediaries pay Part A claims and also conduct reviews and hearings when payment is in dispute.

Carriers perform the same function for Part B claims and also track beneficiaries' out-of-pocket expenses up to the Part B deductible. They also conduct reviews and hearings on Part B claims.

The Second Hurdle: Staying In

People have the idea that they are supposed to stay in the hospital until they are completely well. The simple fact is that Medicare never intended this. Medicare intended to pay for hospitalization only as long as it is medically necessary—that is, as long as the hospital is the only place you could receive the needed care. Most hospital patients are able to be discharged to a skilled nursing facility, to home health care or to their homes after relatively short stays. Medicare does not pay for the nonmedical care of people who have limited ability to care for themselves unless their conditions can be expected to improve with further medical treatment.

Not needing hospital care does not mean that you are completely well. It is likely that you will go home from the hospital needing some further recuperation. As we discussed in chapter 5, it is important to find out how well you can be and to make realistic plans within those limits. Being told that you are ready to be discharged should not be a crisis if you have discussed your situation with your doctor or have asked relatives to make provisions for your postdischarge care.

The same logic and the same procedures that we discussed above under *getting in* apply to *staying in.* Here we discuss the few differences for each of the following:

- Your doctor
- The hospital's utilization review committee
- Medicare+Choice plans
- Your employee or retiree health plan reviewer
- The peer review organization

Your Doctor

Discuss discharge plans with your doctor before you go into the hospital, or as soon as possible after admission, in an emergency or urgent situation. You should ask what course your care is likely to take, what might go wrong, what limitations on your ability to care for yourself you can expect after your hospitalization and what plans you should be making for discharge. Asking these questions puts you in control of the process to some extent.

The Hospital's Utilization Review Committee

The hospital's URC review of your case has no effect on Medicare *unless* the PRO has delegated review of continued hospital stays to it. If you receive a notice that your continued stay in the hospital is no longer needed, you have the right to request a reconsideration and to appeal if the reconsideration is not favorable. The last part of this chapter explains how.

Medicare+Choice Plans

Your Medicare+Choice plan has the right to review your need for continued hospitalization and may recommend that you be discharged. Before it does so, it must issue you a Notice of Noncoverage telling you what your rights are to appeal. You have the right to request an immediate PRO review if you believe you are being discharged from the hospital prematurely. You may also ask your plan to conduct an immediate review; however, there is some financial risk in exercising this option.

Appealing to the PRO affords you financial protection until the PRO issues its decision. Your protection is the same as someone enrolled in original Medicare. You may remain in the hospital until noon of the calendar day following the day the PRO notifies you of its decision.

But filing a request for an **expedited review** with your plan affords you no such financial protection. You are liable for all costs if you lose your appeal. For this reason, we strongly advise you to appeal directly to the PRO.

Your Employee or Retiree Health Plan Reviewer

Just as is the case with admission, a decision by your employee or retiree health plan reviewer that hospital care is not needed has no effect on Medicare as long as the care you need is covered by Medicare and is medically necessary. A finding by your employee health plan reviewer should alert you to the possibility that the PRO or the hospital's URC may find that your continued stay in the hospital is not medically necessary. Again, you should discuss the situation with your doctor and make plans for discharge if he does not seriously disagree with the reviewer.

The Peer Review Organization

One of the jobs of the PRO is to review cases of extended hospital stays. This review can be triggered in a number of ways. See the end of this chapter for instructions on how to appeal a decision not to pay for more time in the hospital.

The PRO's decision affects Medicare's payment for your hospital stay in the following way: You can stay in the hospital until the third day following the date you received the notice that your continued stay was no longer necessary. If you do not request a reconsideration, Medicare will cease payment on the third day following the notice. If you do request reconsideration and get a favorable ruling at any stage of the process, Medicare will pay for time spent in the hospital up until you are discharged or die. If you lose the appeal, you or your insurer must pay for any time spent in the hospital after the PRO rules against you.

Be aware, however, that if you request an *expedited* reconsideration of the PRO's decision, it *may* come before the two days to which you would otherwise be entitled have passed. The moral of the story is that you should not request an expedited reconsideration unless you have made reasonable plans for posthospital care in the event you lose.

The Effect of the Diagnosis-Related Groups System

As stated earlier, the only limit on your hospital stay is its medical necessity. You *cannot* be discharged for any of the following reasons:

- Because your care has cost more than the money amount of your DRG
- Because you have been in the hospital more days than the number of days assigned to your DRG
- Because your hospital has not requested outlier payments
- Because your hospital has not received outlier payments

Only medical necessity should govern your length of stay. When you go into the hospital, you are supposed to receive a notice telling you that you cannot be discharged "because your DRG has run out." A copy is shown on pages 152-153.

Making Sure Your Care Is Adequate

Making sure that you receive adequate care in the hospital is a subject that is beyond the scope of this book. There is, in fact, a book devoted exclusively to this subject: *Take This Book to the Hospital With You,* by Charles B. Inlander and Ed Weiner. We suggest that you read it. It contains valuable advice for any hospital stay, whether or not Medicare pays for it.

There is a temptation for hospitals to provide less than adequate care to Medicare beneficiaries. First, they are afraid that your care will cost more than the DRG for your condition(s) will pay. Second, they are afraid that they will not be able to maximize the profit they could make on the DRG. Right now economic reality for hospitals is that they can make the most money by admitting you and then giving you minimal care. This is the situation the PROs were set up to police. There are perverse incentives in any payment system, and the DRG system is better, from a number of angles, than the pay-for-each-day system that preceded it.

The key point to remember is that your status as a Medicare patient should make no difference. Hospitals make about 50 percent of their revenues from Medicare patients. The hospital needs you as much as you need it.

All this assumes, of course, that you know what good care is. This is something about which lay opinions have been disregarded in the past. Another way to make sure your care is adequate is to be aware of your **consumer protections**. Congress has mandated that Medicare beneficiaries have full protection under the law, but the problem is that neither Congress or Medicare has defined full protection. The closest attempt to date is the **Patients' Bill of Rights** found in appendix C.

Controlling the Doctors

All the controversy about hospitals and Medicare makes us forget that it is ultimately the doctors who control the hospital, at least as far as medical care is concerned. There is a good deal of self-doubt in the profession about the way things are done now. You can see a wide sampling in *Medicine on Trial*, by Charles B. Inlander, Lowell Levin and Ed Weiner. The material covered in that book is beyond the scope of this one.

We do want to mention one thing to watch out for, something that doctors regret but feel they can't control: the clinical "cascade." What happens is this: You go in for a relatively simple treatment, and you have a bad reaction to the dye used in a test or something else does not go exactly according to your doctor's original plan. He asks a specialist to examine you. The specialist treats you for the bad reaction to the dye but thinks she spots something else, so she orders some tests. They show a possible abnormality, you're in the hospital, so it might as well be checked out now, and . . .

All too soon you are the recipient of as much medical attention as the hospital can muster, being treated for reactions to treatments that were

continued on page 154

AN IMPORTANT MESSAGE FROM MEDICARE

YOUR RIGHTS WHILE YOU ARE A MEDICARE HOSPITAL PATIENT

- You have the right to receive all the hospital care that is necessary for the proper diagnosis and treatment of your illness or injury. According to federal law, your discharge date must be determined solely by your medical needs, not by Diagnosis-Related Groups (DRG) or Medicare payments.

- You have the right to be fully informed about decisions affecting your Medicare coverage and payment for your hospital stay and for any posthospital services.

- You have the right to request a review by a Peer Review Organization (PRO) of any written Notice of Noncoverage that you receive from the hospital stating that Medicare will no longer pay for your hospital care.

TALK WITH YOUR DOCTOR ABOUT YOUR STAY IN THE HOSPITAL

You and your doctor know more about your condition and your health needs than anyone else. Decisions about your medical treatment should be made between you and your doctor. If you have any questions about your medical treatment, your need for continued hospital care, your discharge or your need for possible posthospital care, don't hesitate to ask your doctor. The hospital's patient representative or social worker will also help you with your questions and concerns about hospital services.

IF YOU THINK YOU ARE BEING ASKED TO LEAVE THE HOSPITAL TOO SOON

- Ask a hospital representative for a written notice of explanation immediately if you have not already received one. This notice is called a Notice of Noncoverage. You must have this Notice of Noncoverage if you wish to exercise your right to request a review by the PRO.

- The Notice of Noncoverage states that either your doctor or the PRO agrees with the hospital's decision that Medicare will no longer pay for your hospital care.
  + If the hospital and your doctor agree, the PRO does not review your case before a Notice of Noncoverage is issued. But the PRO will respond to your request for a review of your Notice of Noncoverage and seek your opinion. You cannot be made to pay for your hospital care until the PRO makes its decision if you request the review by noon of the first workday after you receive the Notice of Noncoverage.
  + If the hospital and your doctor disagree, the hospital may request the PRO to review your case. If it does make such a request, the hospital is required to send you a notice to that effect. In this situation the PRO must agree with the hospital, or the hospital cannot issue a Notice of Noncoverage. You may request that the PRO reconsider your case after you receive a Notice of Noncoverage, but since the PRO has already reviewed your case once, you may have to pay for at least one day of hospital care before the PRO completes this reconsideration.

IF YOU DO NOT REQUEST A REVIEW, THE HOSPITAL MAY BILL YOU FOR ALL THE COSTS OF YOUR STAY BEGINNING WITH THE THIRD DAY AFTER YOU RECEIVE THE NOTICE OF NONCOVERAGE. THE HOSPITAL, HOWEVER, CANNOT CHARGE YOU FOR CARE UNLESS IT PROVIDES YOU WITH A NOTICE OF NONCOVERAGE.

HOW TO REQUEST A REVIEW OF THE NOTICE OF NONCOVERAGE

- If the Notice of Noncoverage states that your physician agrees with the hospital's decision:
    + You must make your request for review to the PRO by noon of the first calendar day after you receive the Notice of Noncoverage by contacting the PRO by phone or in writing.
    + The PRO must ask for your views about your case before making its decision. The PRO will inform you by phone and in writing of its decision on the review.
    + If the PRO agrees with the Notice of Noncoverage, you may be billed for all costs of your stay beginning at noon of the day after you receive the PRO's decision.
    + Thus, you will not be responsible for the cost of hospital care before you receive the PRO's decision.
- If the Notice of Noncoverage states that the PRO agrees with the hospital's decision:
    + You should make your request for reconsideration to the PRO immediately upon receipt of the Notice of Noncoverage by contacting the PRO by phone or in writing.
    + The PRO can take up to three calendar days from receipt of your request to complete the review. The PRO will inform you in writing of its decision on the review.
    + Since the PRO has already reviewed your case once, prior to the issuance of the Notice of Noncoverage, the hospital is permitted to begin billing you for the cost of your stay beginning with the third calendar day after you receive your Notice of Noncoverage even if the PRO has not completed its review.
    + Thus, if the PRO continues to agree with the Notice of Noncoverage, you may have to pay for at least one day of hospital care.

NOTE: The process described above is called **immediate review**. If you miss the deadline for this immediate review while you are in the hospital, you may still request a review of Medicare's decision to no longer pay for your care at any point during your hospital stay or after you have left the hospital. The Notice of Noncoverage will tell you how to request this review.

POSTHOSPITAL CARE

When your doctor determines that you no longer need all the specialized services provided in a hospital but you still require medical care, he or she may discharge you to a skilled nursing facility or home care. The discharge planner at the hospital will help arrange for the services you may need after your discharge. Medicare and supplemental insurance policies have limited coverage for skilled nursing facility care and home health care. Therefore, you should find out which services will or will not be covered and how payment will be made. Consult with your doctor, hospital discharge planner, patient representative and your family in making preparations for care after you leave the hospital. Don't hesitate to ask questions.

ACKNOWLEDGMENT OF RECEIPT—My signature only acknowledges my receipt of this message from [name of hospital] on [date] and does not waive any of my rights to request a review or make me liable for any payment.

_____   _____
Signature of beneficiary or   Date of receipt
person acting on behalf of beneficiary

given because you had reactions to other treatments, with your admitting doctor somewhere in the background, peering over the shoulders of the specialists and house staff who surround you.

The only one who can stop this is *you,* sad to say. You should question every treatment and insist on knowing, at every moment, which doctor is primarily responsible for your care. You should negotiate for assignment with every doctor who treats you. If you need to ask whether or not you will be billed for a service, do so. Refuse it if the doctor will not take assignment, and ask whoever is in charge of your case to find someone who will.

If you are too ill to deal with this, we suggest that you give someone you trust, and who is willing to steer your care, a durable power of attorney. This was discussed at considerable length in chapter 5. A durable power of attorney will enable that trusted person to handle these matters for you.

Remember:

- You have a right to the same quality medical care as anyone else the hospital serves.

- You have the right to refuse services you do not want.

- You have the right to leave the hospital, even against medical advice.

Patient Self-Determination Act

You have the right to make decisions about your care, including the right to refuse it. Because many people were unaware that they had this right, Congress passed the Patient Self-Determination Act. This law requires providers to advise patients of their right to make patient care decisions. The law includes the following provisions:

- All adult individuals must be provided with written information about their rights under state law to make health care decisions, including the right to accept or refuse treatment and the right to execute advance directives.

- The descriptions of state law will be developed at the state level, through state agencies, associations or other private, not-for-profit entities. The federal law also does not override any state law that would allow a health care provider to object on the basis of conscience to implementing an advance directive.

- Hospitals, nursing facilities and hospices must provide the written information at the time of the individual's admission.

- Home health or personal care services must provide the written information prior to providing care.

- Medicare- and Medicaid-certified prepaid health plans such as HMOs must provide the written information upon enrollment.

- The provider must document in the patient's medical record whether she has signed an advance directive.

- The provider must not discriminate against an individual based on whether he has executed an advance directive.

- The provider must provide staff and community education on advance directives. (See page 137 for more information.)

Reconsideration and Appeals

This section covers how to obtain reconsideration of the following:

- Decisions about hospital care by the PROs
- Decisions about payment for hospital care by intermediaries

Peer Review Organization Decisions

The PRO is involved in determining whether or not Medicare will:

- Pay for your hospital admission
- Pay for your continued stay in the hospital
- Pay for your admission to a skilled nursing facility
- Pay for your continued stay in a skilled nursing facility
- Pay for an outpatient procedure to be done in the hospital
- Require a second opinion before paying for surgery

Key Points:

- In all your dealings with the PROs, there are only two issues: (1) the *medical necessity* of your being cared for at all and (2) the *medical necessity* of your being cared for *in the way your doctor wants to care for you.* All other issues are extraneous. Stay focused on these points.

- There is a great deal of uncertainty in medicine. It is unlikely that what your doctor wants to do is totally unreasonable. You and he should emphasize *why* it is acceptable as good medical care.

- Keep copies of everything you send to the PRO. It is advisable to send materials *certified mail, return receipt requested.* This gives you proof of the date you mailed material and the date on which the PRO (or other recipient of your papers such as your Social Security office) received it.

- If you are dealing with a decision that your continued stay is no longer medically necessary, make sure you understand when Medicare will no longer pay for your hospital stay.

- A PRO review of care that you have already had rarely requires you to pay for it. You cannot retroactively be required to pay for care you've already received unless you can reasonably be expected to have known that it wasn't covered. (See chapter 3 for more information on this.)

Procedure

The procedure that follows is generic. It applies to all actions by the PROs. Only the evidence submitted would differ.

Notices: Your denial is called a Notice of Noncoverage, and it will explain why something is being denied.

If you receive such a notice *while you are in the hospital,* it's important to understand that there are two tracks and different results possible: First, if you are asking the PRO to review the hospital's decision, you are not responsible for services received before you get the notice of the PRO's decision. Second, if you are asking the PRO to rethink its own decision, the hospital may start billing you beginning with the third calendar day after you received the Notice of Noncoverage. If the PRO does not reverse its position and you decide not to stay in the hospital, you may have to pay for the third day. If you decide to stay, you are responsible for the further cost of your care.

How to Appeal (Request a Reconsideration of) a Peer Review Organization Decision: You can appeal the decision of the PRO by filing a request for reconsideration with the PRO itself at the address for the PRO shown on the notice you received, at any Social Security office or at a Railroad Retirement office if you are a Railroad Retirement beneficiary.

Your doctor and the hospital also have the right to file an appeal. They do *not* have the right that you have to an expedited reconsideration.

Time to File the Request for Reconsideration: You must file your request for reconsideration within 60 days of the date you receive the Notice of Noncoverage. Unless you can prove otherwise, the notice is deemed to have been received by you five days after the date on it. (For example, the notice is dated January 5. You are deemed to have received it on January 10 unless you can prove you received it later. Your 60-day period for appeal started on January 10. The last day you can file an appeal is March 10, the 60th day after the deemed receipt of the notice.) Some examples of how the dates run are provided below. You can file this request with the PRO or at your Social Security office or Railroad Retirement office if you are a Railroad Retirement beneficiary.

Sample Time Periods for Filing Requests for Reconsideration		
NOTICE OF NONCOVERAGE MAILED	DEEMED RECEIVED	LAST DAY TO FILE REQUEST
January 5	January 10	March 10
March 15	March 20	May 20
November 27	December 1	January 29 (of next year)

Request for Extension of Time to File: If you need more than 60 days to file your appeal, you can request more time at any Social Security office or Railroad Retirement office. You cannot file an extension request with an intermediary. You will be notified in writing of the time granted to you.

"Good Cause" for Late Filing: Generally, you will be allowed to file late if there is what the PRO considers to be "good cause" for it. The regulations are very broad, and it is hard to see what exactly might be considered good cause. The regulations give examples such as serious illness, a death in the family, failure to receive information you had requested before the 60-day limit, a misunderstanding of what the PRO notice told you and so on.

Obtaining Information: Both you and your doctor have a right to see the information on which the PRO based its decision. You should ask for this when you file your request for reconsideration. You may add to the information anything you or your doctor want to add.

Expedited Reconsideration and Time Limits: You can request that the PRO make an expedited review or reconsideration of the denial. How fast "expedited" has to be depends on the circumstances:

- Within three calendar days if you are still a patient in the hospital and you receive a Notice of Noncoverage

- Within three calendar days if the initial determination was a pre-admission denial of hospital care

- Within 10 calendar days if you are in a skilled nursing facility

- Within 30 calendar days if you are appealing a hospital's decision not to admit you because it believes your proposed stay will not be covered by Medicare and in every situation in which someone other than you files the appeal. Having expedited redetermination available is a very important reason for you to file the appeal and have the doctor or hospital submit information as part of an appeal.

Notices and Appeals: When the PRO provides you with its reconsideration decision, it must do so *in writing* and inform you of the following:

- The decision

- The reasons for it

- A statement of the effect the decision has on what Medicare will pay for or has paid for

- A statement of your appeal rights, with complete instructions for filing the appeal

When you receive a notice of a reconsideration decision that is not in your favor, consider whether you want to request a hearing. A hearing is more formal than a reconsideration, and it entitles you to appear before an administrative law judge. If you do request a hearing, it is wise to have a lawyer involved. Hearings can involve subpoenaing witnesses and other legal steps. A hearing is less formal than a court case but far more formal than a request for reconsideration. To make it easier on the beneficiary, Medicare is attempting to transact more and more business over the phone—including hearings. Our advice is this: Although a hearing can be conducted over the phone, you should carefully consider appearing in person. It is sometimes easier—and more effective— to make your case in person, depending on the circumstances.

Only you, not your doctor or the hospital, have the right to request a hearing. The rules for filing a request for a hearing are exactly the same as for filing for reconsideration with the PRO—60 days, counted from five days after the date of the notice. Follow the instructions on the information you receive with the PRO's Notice of Reconsideration.

You may request a hearing only if the amount in dispute is $100 or more.

The first thing the administrative law judge will attempt to determine is whether the controversy involves at least $100 (with the price of health care these days, it almost surely will). If the administrative law judge determines that the amount is less than $100, he will notify you and any other concerned parties that he has determined this and that you and concerned parties have 15 days to show why he is wrong. If no evidence is submitted within 15 days, the request for a hearing is dismissed. (You will not have to worry about this if you don't receive such a notice.)

You will be notified by the judge of the date of the hearing at least 10 days before it is scheduled.

If the judge's decision is unfavorable, you can appeal to the Social Security Appeals Council. Your attorney can tell you how to do this. The Appeals Council does not take all the appeals addressed to it. If $1,000 or more is at issue, you can appeal an Appeals Council decision (or the judge's decision if the Appeals Council refused a hearing) to the federal courts. This must be done within 60 days of the date of the Appeals Council decision on your case or its decision not to hear it.

Requesting Reconsideration on Payment by Intermediaries

The procedures in this section apply to denial of payment for all services other than doctors' services after you have left the hospital. They also apply to notices regarding hospital care that you receive from the Medicare intermediary while you are in the hospital.

Notices: Your denial will come either in the form of a Medicare Summary Notice (MSN) or in the form of a letter. In any case it must be in writing. It will explain the reason that something is being denied. A typical MSN is shown on pages 78-79.

How to Appeal (Request a Reconsideration of) a Payment Denial or Intermediary Determination That Care Is Not Medically Necessary: You can appeal the intermediary's decision by filing a request for reconsideration with the intermediary itself at the address shown on the MSN, at any Social Security office or at a Railroad Retirement office if you are a Railroad Retirement beneficiary.

Your doctor and the hospital have the right to file an appeal only if you do not plan to do so and you certify this in writing on a form they will provide. They do *not* have the right that you have to an expedited reconsideration.

Time to File the Request for Reconsideration: You must file your request for reconsideration within 60 days of the date you are notified of the denial. Unless you can prove otherwise, the notice is deemed to have been received by you five days after the date on it. (For example, the notice is dated January 5. You are deemed to have received it on January 10 unless you can prove you received it later. Your 60-day period for appeal started on January 10. The last day you can file an appeal is March 10, the 60th day after the deemed receipt of the notice.)

Request for Extension of Time to File: If you need more than 60 days to file your appeal, you can request more time at any Social Security office or Railroad Retirement office. You cannot file an extension request with an intermediary. You will be notified in writing of the time granted you.

"Good Cause" for Late Filing: Generally, you will be allowed to file late if there is what the intermediary considers to be "good cause" for it. The regulations are very broad, and it is hard to see what exactly might be considered good cause. The regulations give examples such as serious illness, a death in the family, failure to receive information you had requested before the 60-day limit, a misunderstanding of what the intermediary notice told you and so on.

Obtaining Information: Both you and your doctor have a right to see the information on which the intermediary based its decision. You should ask for this when you file your request for reconsideration. You may add to the information anything you or your doctor want to add.

Expedited Reconsideration: There is a procedure for expedited appeals under Part A (hospital insurance), but it may be used only if both the person appealing and the Secretary of Health and Human Services agree that the only issue is a constitutional one. This is a rare situation.

What to Include: Use HCFA Form 2649—*Request for Reconsideration of a Part A Health Insurance Benefit*—to file your request for reconsideration on a Part A claim.

You can request an appeal with just a letter, but using the form ensures that you include everything that is needed. You should ask your doctor to provide medical documentation. It is important for both you and your doctor to focus on the issue at hand and not to editorialize. The general issues you will be dealing with are the medical necessity of the service, whether Medicare covers it, whether you are entitled to it and whether the amount paid is what ought to have been paid. Medical necessity issues boil down to appropriate medical judgment. Your doctor will probably want to submit information regarding your condition, plus evidence from the medical literature that indicates that what the intermediary wants is unwise.

Time Limits: The regulations provide no time limit for a decision on a Part A request for reconsideration.

Notices and Appeals: When the intermediary provides you with its decision, it must do so *in writing* and inform you of the following:

- The decision

- The reasons for it

- A statement of the effect the decision has on what Medicare will pay for or has paid for

- A statement of your appeal rights, with complete instructions for filing the appeal

When you receive a notice of a reconsideration decision that is not in your favor, consider whether you want to request a hearing. A hearing is more formal than a reconsideration and entitles you to appear before an administrative law judge. If you do request a hearing, it is wise to have a lawyer involved. Hearings can involve subpoenaing witnesses and other legal steps. A hearing is less formal than a court case but far more formal than a request for reconsideration.

Only you, not your doctor or the hospital, have the right to request a hearing. The rules for filing a request for a hearing are exactly the same as for filing for reconsideration—60 days, counted from five days after the date of the notice. You should file your request for a hearing on HCFA Form 501.1 unless the information you received with the Notice of Reconsideration tells you to do something else.

You may request a hearing only if the amount in dispute is $100 or more.

As we said before, the first thing the administrative law judge will attempt to determine is whether the controversy involves at least $100. If the judge determines that the amount is less than $100, he will notify you and any other concerned parties that he has determined this and that you and concerned parties have 15 days to show why he is wrong. If no evidence is submitted within 15 days, the request for a hearing is dismissed. (You will not have to worry about this if you don't receive such a notice.)

You will be notified by the administrative law judge of the date of the hearing at least 10 days before it is scheduled.

If the judge's decision is unfavorable, you can appeal to the Social Security Appeals Council. Your attorney can tell you how to do this. The Appeals Council does not take all the appeals addressed to it. If $1,000 or more is at issue, you can appeal an Appeals Council decision (or the judge's decision if the Appeals Council refused a hearing) to the federal courts. This must be done within 60 days of the date of the Appeals Council determination or its decision not to hear your case.

If you receive a favorable determination, Medicare pays its usual amounts for the services rendered. If you do not receive a favorable determination, you pay.

Appealing Decisions Made by Carriers on Part B Claims

Most of this chapter dealt with the appeals procedure for PROs and intermediaries because they handle most hospital inpatient decisions. However, because much of the care you receive in the hospital is provided by doctors, we need to review the procedures for appealing decisions about payments to doctors as well.

You also have the right to appeal decisions involving services covered under Part B of Medicare. This may include the request for a service, payment for a service or the decision not to pay for a service. If you disagree with the decision made by the carrier, you may appeal—following the information printed on the MSN—and you must do so within the time frame listed.

How to Appeal (Request a Reconsideration of) a Payment or Service Denial by a Carrier

Use the following forms to make your appeal.

- HCFA Form 1964—*Request for Reconsideration on Part B Claims*
- HCFA Form 1965—*Request for Hearing on Part B Claims*

You never have to use these forms, but using them will help you record all the information you need. You can also send a letter. Here is the procedure:

- You write to the carrier and ask for a reconsideration of the decision.

- You have six months from the date the decision was made (the expiration date is printed on the MSN).

- You can mail or hand deliver your request to the carrier or contact any Social Security office or Railroad Retirement office if you are a Railroad Retirement beneficiary.

- The carrier will send you a notice advising you of its decision.

If you disagree with the carrier's reconsideration decision, you may request a hearing before the carrier's hearing officer. You have six months from the date of the carrier's decision to file your request for a hearing. Use HCFA Form 1965 or a letter to request your hearing. You will receive a decision from the carrier's hearing officer advising you of its decision.

If you disagree with the carrier's hearing officer, you may request a hearing before an administrative law judge if your claim involves at least $500. You have 60 days from the date you receive the carrier's decision to request a hearing.

The judge will notify you of his decision. If it's in your favor, Medicare will cover the service. If the decision is not in your favor, you may appeal to the Social Security Appeals Council; however, the Appeals Council does not take every case that is addressed to it. If $1,000 or more is at issue and you disagree with the decision made by the judge and Appeals Council, you can appeal to the federal courts.

Appealing Decisions Made by Medicare+Choice Plans

For all service-related requests, a Medicare+Choice plan *must* make the initial determination within 14 calendar days. You may also request a 72-hour expedited review if any delay in care would be detrimental to your health. Under original Medicare, reviews are generally done *after* you've had a service. Under managed care, however, there's a certain urgency because treatment decisions are made *before* you have the service. For this reason, Medicare requires that all requests for treatment be decided "as expeditiously as the enrollee's health condition requires."

Notices and Appeals: When the Medicare+Choice plan provides you with its decision, it must do so in *writing* and inform you of the following:

- The reason for it

- Your right to either a standard or expedited reconsideration

- A description of both the standard and expedited review processes

- A description of the rest of the appeals process with complete instructions for filing your appeal

If you are dissatisfied with the initial determination made by your Medicare+Choice plan, you have the right to request a reconsideration. The request for reconsideration is the first step in the appeals process.

A standard reconsideration must be completed within 30 calendar days, and an expedited reconsideration must be done within 72 hours.

If your plan, on reconsideration, confirms its initial determination not to approve your request for services or pay a claim, your case is sent to the Center for Health Dispute Resolution (CHDR). The CHDR renders its decision within 30 calendar days or within 72 hours if an expedited review is requested.

If the CHDR doesn't approve your request, you may take your appeal to an administrative law judge of the Social Security Administration. You may request a hearing if the amount in dispute is $100 or more.

If the judge's decision is unfavorable, you may request that the Appeals Council of the Social Security Administration review the judge's decision.

Finally, you may file suit in federal court if the amount in dispute is $1,000 or more.

Knowing your rights and when to exercise them is the first step in being a fully informed Medicare beneficiary.

In this chapter you will learn: What Medicare covers under skilled nursing care ▪ How Medicaid can help pay for nursing home care ▪ What to look for when selecting long-term-care insurance ▪ How to evaluate a nursing home ▪ What home health care services are covered

7. Nursing Homes, Home Health Care and Medicare

The nursing home business is a $70-billion-per-year industry. Of the nation's 37 million citizens ages 65 and above, 1.5 million (4 percent) live in nursing homes. The average cost of a year's stay is $27,500. The average stay, 838 days, costs $62,850. The average charge is around $75 per day. The Brookings Institution, a Washington think tank, estimates that by the year 2018, almost 8 percent of the elderly will live in nursing homes, at an annual cost of $55,000 per person.

Nursing Homes Are Partially Covered

We explained in chapter 3 that Medicare does not, as many people think, pay for what we usually think of as "nursing home care." As you may recall, there are three levels of nursing home care:

▪ *Skilled nursing facilities* offer care delivered by registered and licensed practical nurses on the orders of attending physicians. They offer services such as oxygen therapy; intravenous and tube feedings; care of catheters and wound drains; and physical, occupational and speech therapy.

- *Intermediate care facilities* provide less intensive care than skilled nursing facilities. Patients are generally more mobile, and rehabilitation therapies are stressed.

- *Custodial, or sheltered, care* is nonmedical. Residents do not require constant attention from nurses and aides but need assistance with one or more daily activities or no longer want to be bothered with keeping up a house. The social needs of residents are met in a secure environment free of as many anxieties as possible.

Medicare covers nursing home care at the skilled nursing facility level only. Further, Medicare pays for skilled nursing facility services *only* if the following conditions are met:

- The nursing home must be a skilled nursing facility and certified to participate in the Medicare program.

- A three-day prior hospitalization is required, and a physician must certify that the person requires skilled care.

- There must be ongoing utilization review to determine if the person is receiving skilled nursing services.

- If a determination is made that skilled care is no longer required, Medicare coverage ceases.

You should be aware that Medicare is not a long-term solution to paying for nursing home care because it does not cover intermediate or custodial (sheltered) care, the two most common levels of care required, and its coverage for skilled nursing facility care is limited to 100 days per benefit period. Medicare pays all costs for the first 20 days; however, you are responsible for a copayment from the 21st through the 100th day. See page 46 for the skilled nursing facility benefit period and costs. Let's consider an example:

> *The Smith family's aged grandmother, Iphigenia, had a stroke, fell and broke her hip. She had to have the hip replaced with an artificial one and has been in and out of the hospital with infections and failure of the bone to solidify around the hip. The last stay in the hospital seems to have finally fixed her hip, but she is currently unable to walk, has trouble with bowel and bladder control and tends to get dehydrated very easily. She needs a long stay in a nursing home for recuperation, with almost constant nursing attention to ensure that her wound does not get reinfected and her fluid intake is adequate, and to get occupational and speech therapy. As things turn out, she has to stay in the nursing home for an entire year after her last discharge from the hospital.*

Let's see what Medicare paid: The nursing home charged $100 per day for skilled nursing facility services. (This figure included the room charge plus estimated ancillary charges for items such as medicine and equipment.) Medicare paid for the first 20 days and all costs above $96 for days 21 through 100. That leaves 265 days to pay for.

What's the portion paid by Medicare, and what's the portion paid by the Smiths?

Total cost: $100 × 365 =	$36,500
Medicare payment for first 20 days:	
20 × $100 =	$ 2,000
Smiths' copayment for days 21-100:	
80 × $96 =	$ 7,680
Medicare payment for days 21-100:	
80 × $4 ($100 − $96) =	$ 320
Smiths' payment for days 101-365:	
265 × $100 =	$26,500
Medicare paid:	$ 2,320 (6%)
The Smiths paid:	$34,180 (94%)

Another common misconception is that "Medicare will take care of you until you're well." This is not true. Most Medicare recipients recover sufficiently to leave the hospital, but they are discharged when they no longer need hospital services—not when they are completely well. Some never get completely well. Some never recover sufficiently to leave a skilled nursing facility. In recognition of this, Medicare imposes a cutoff point for skilled nursing facility services. Longer-term needs are taken care of by federal/state programs such as Medicaid and **Supplemental Security Income**. There is a growing recognition on the part of the policy makers that some of the needs of the elderly such as help with eating and dressing are not medical needs. They're not medical because medicine can't do anything for them. They are social problems that ought to be handled outside the medical model. The federal government has approved **social health maintenance organizations (SHMOs)** as a way to provide care outside the medical model, but this sort of work is still in its infancy. For the moment, don't assume that Medicare will take care of every need you have for long-term care. It won't.

Medical necessity is *the* key issue in payment for skilled nursing facility services. The skilled nursing facility regulations go to great lengths to define what is and is not skilled nursing facility care. The key is that care complex enough to require the services of a nurse or skilled rehabilitation personnel is covered; care that you could do yourself is not. But complications may require skilled-nursing-facility-level care, even for situations that would normally not be covered. Basically, skilled nursing facility care is rehabilitation; if your condition cannot be expected to improve as a result of skilled nursing facility care *and* you do not need observation by skilled personnel, your care will not be covered. Obviously, what your doctor writes in the chart makes a big difference in what gets covered. If you are worried about coverage of skilled nursing facility services, discuss this with your doctor.

Do You Really Need a Nursing Home?

It is true, of course, that some older people are crippled by arthritis, have Alzheimer's disease or have another form of senile dementia that makes it impossible for them to live without constant supervision; others have problems that require constant, round-the-clock custodial care. These people account for only about 5 percent of the elderly. (There are, of course, others who are cared for by a spouse or other relative.) The majority of the over-65 population seems to do quite well without nursing home care.

In our experience, many older people think they need nursing home care because they are no longer able to do one or a few of the things they did when they were young. If you are no longer able to drive, this does not mean you need a nursing home—it means you need transportation. If you are unable to cook, this does not mean you need a nursing home—it means you need someone to prepare meals for you. Most of the elderly face difficulties that are no more severe than those faced by younger handicapped people who are able to live independently.

Part of the reason many older people think they need a nursing home if they are no longer able to do everything they used to do is that they share society's prejudice against the aged. A handicap heroically overcome in a 35-year-old is an infirmity that demands nursing home care in a 65-year-old—or so people think. In chapter 5 we discussed some of these prejudices as they affect your dealings with your doctor. We suggest you reread the section "The Doctor's Obligation to Inform You Fully" again. Are you, perhaps, prejudiced against the elderly yourself?

The Health Status Checklist on page 170 will help you assess the level of care that you (or an aged relative) need. In using it, think very carefully about the person's level of functioning. If you're not sure, put a question mark. On items with a question mark, you may want to seek some professional advice in evaluating the person's capabilities.

Caring for a bedridden, elderly person can be a full-time job. The caregiver must be on the lookout for the development of pressure sores (decubitus ulcers), incontinence, dehydration, malnutrition, development of contractures (flexion and fixation of a joint caused by shortening of the muscles) from too little limb movement and the unusual drug reactions that are common in the elderly.

For those who are not bedridden, adult day care, home health care, homemaker services, sharing a home with other elderly people, Meals on Wheels, shopping services and adult foster care may be alternatives that prevent the need for nursing homes. For the availability of these services, you can check with your local Area Agency on Aging, the medical social services office of the hospital (if the person is in the hospital awaiting discharge) and the state department of social services. Many are listed in the telephone book under the "Guide to Human Services" section.

Paying for Custodial Care in a Nursing Home

As we have seen, Medicare does not cover care in a nursing home that is custodial, or nonmedical, in nature. Two alternatives may help you pay for custodial care if you really need it: Medicaid and private nursing home insurance.

Medicaid

The Medicaid program provides medical care for the poor. It was tacked onto the Medicare bill at the last possible second, and its passage by Congress, together with Medicare, amazed its advocates. The program still shows the features of its hasty design. Medicaid is intended for the very poor who have nowhere else to turn, but not all of the very poor are covered.

You are *automatically* eligible for Medicaid if you are eligible for, or are receiving, Supplemental Security Income payments for aged, blind and disabled, but you must apply at a state welfare office. If you meet the requirements for Supplemental Security Income, there is little chance

Health Status Checklist*

Read each statement *very carefully* before deciding if it applies to the person in question, then place a check mark in front of those that describe the person's conditions. Think in terms of *"Does this person have difficulty with"*:

_____ 1. *Bathing*—requires assistance from another person

_____ 2. *Continence*—difficulty controlling the bladder or bowels

_____ 3. *Dressing*—either requires assistance or does not dress at all

_____ 4. *Eating*—requires assistance, either from another person or via tube or intravenously

_____ 5. *Mobility*—either requires the assistance from another person to walk or is confined to a chair or bed

_____ 6. *Using toilet room*—either requires assistance from another person or does not use one at all

_____ 7. *Speech*—either completely lost or is so severely impaired that it can be understood only with difficulty. In other words, the person cannot carry on a normal conversation.

_____ 8. *Hearing*—either completely lost or is so severely impaired that only a few words a person says or loud noises can be heard

_____ 9. *Vision*—either blind or is so severely impaired that television cannot be seen 8 to 12 feet away. Features of a familiar person can be recognized within 2 to 3 feet.

_____ 10. *Mental status*—cannot understand (or remember) simple instruction; requires constant supervision or restraints for his own safety

*Suggested by the Department of Health and Human Services, Long-Term-Care Survey.

that you would have to give up additional income or assets to qualify for Medicaid.

If your income, less certain deductions and medical bills, is within certain (low) limits, you may be eligible for Medicaid as **medically needy**. You must "spend down" to pay medical bills to the point at which you are eligible; after that, Medicaid pays for medical bills as long as you are eligible.

Medicaid is a state-run program that receives federal funds. States make most of the rules, and the trend in recent years has been to make the Medicaid requirements more stringent. Because these strict requirements forced many couples into poverty, Congress enacted new rules designed to limit impoverishment of the at-home spouse. Under these rules, the at-home spouse retains certain assets for living expenses, and half of the assets help to pay for the nursing home care of the other spouse. In this situation, Medicaid doesn't pay the entire cost of care, and the at-home spouse isn't driven into poverty.

Here are some provisions of the legislation:

- In any month in which a married person is in a nursing home, no income of the at-home spouse is to be considered available to the spouse in the nursing home.

- Income is considered the property of the person to whom it is paid. Income paid to both spouses is attributed 50 percent to each.

- The home, household goods and personal effects of both spouses are not counted in considering Medicaid eligibility.

- All assets other than these will be counted and divided in two. If the at-home spouse has less than $16,152, the spouse in the nursing home may transfer assets to him to make up to $16,152 available to the at-home spouse. (States may, at their option, raise this figure to any amount less than $80,760. The $16,152 amount is indexed to inflation.)

- The assets that remain in the name of the spouse in the nursing home are considered available to pay for his nursing home care. All assets in excess of $80,760 are attributed to the spouse in the nursing home and are considered available to pay for nursing home care.

- States must allow nursing home residents to retain certain sums for medical expenses not covered by Medicare or Medicaid before contributing to the expense of their nursing home care. The states may place "reasonable limits" on the amounts spent.

- States must allow the at-home spouse sufficient income from the other spouse to bring total household income of the at-home spouse to at least 150 percent of the federal poverty level for a two-person household. States are not required to allow more than $2,019 per month, except by court order or change in regulation.

The current regulations require that the assets and income of your spouse and your parents be considered in determining your eligibility for Medicaid, with few exceptions. This is a very important point: Your spouse and parents do not *actually* have to give anything toward the cost of your care, but your *eligibility* is determined as though they do. The exact requirements, as well as the amount of assets and income you may retain while still remaining eligible, vary from state to state because of the latitude allowed by the federal government in setting some of the income and assets limits. Check the list of state Medicaid offices in appendix E to find out where to call to determine the exact eligibility requirements for your state.

Medicaid services in some states are more restrictive than Medicare services. If the service you are receiving is covered under Medicare and not Medicaid, Medicaid does not pay the Medicare copayments and deductibles applicable to that service. If the service is covered under both, it will, although there may be additional limits. To find out whether you are eligible for Medicaid, apply at any state welfare office. The welfare office is required to take your application and make a formal determination of eligibility even if you are told that you are not eligible.

When you apply, you should bring proof of age, financial status and any disability you may have. The proof of financial status should include bank statements for checking and savings accounts, rent or mortgage payment receipts, loan papers for your car or the title to it, any documents relating to stock or bond ownership and check stubs for any regular payments you receive. You should also have the amount of your Social Security check if you receive Social Security payments. You should always have your Social Security number. Bring your medical bills, or copies of them, for the past year.

When you call the welfare office to make your appointment, ask what is needed. This will save you a delay in getting your eligibility determined and perhaps avoid another trip.

You can transfer your assets to someone other than your spouse or parents (for example, a child) in order to become eligible for Medicaid, but you must do so within the time frame and manner permitted in your state. In addition, provisions found in the Health Insurance

Portability and Accountability Act of 1996 impose severe penalties on individuals who *knowingly and willfully* dispose of assets in order to qualify for Medicaid. As we've said before, *do not* dispose of any assets until you discuss your situation with a qualified attorney.

The exception to this is the division-of-assets provision designed to protect the financial interests of the at-home spouse. Under it, the spouse who is entering the nursing home can transfer assets up to $15,000 (or higher, if a state elects) to the spouse who is staying at home. Outside this provision, if you want to transfer your assets in order to become eligible for nursing home coverage under Medicaid, *you should do so only with the services of a lawyer who understands the Medicaid program.* This is both to protect you and to ensure that you will be found eligible for Medicaid, based on the action you took. There is no point in transferring assets only to find that you are still not eligible or that your action results in legal action against you or your family.

This translates into what we've said before: *You should explore all other alternatives before deciding to enter a nursing home.*

Private Insurance for Nursing Home Care

A decade ago there were only two companies offering nursing home insurance. Today there are more than 100. Back then many plans had so many limitations that the coverage was practically worthless. Now all that has changed for the better. As a result, the Health Insurance Association of America reported that sales of long-term-care insurance policies have averaged between 400,000 and 500,000 policies per year since 1987. Today some 4.3 million policies are in effect, and even the most conservative projections indicate the growth in sales is expected to continue. With the high cost of nursing home care, purchasing a long-term-care policy could be a very wise investment.

The typical benefits offered by policies include coverage for skilled, intermediate and custodial care; home health care; adult day care; alternate care (living arrangements such as group home or shared residence); and respite care. They are guaranteed renewable, have a 30-day "free look" provision and have a six-month exclusion for preexisting conditions. These are just some of the features you should consider when purchasing a policy. Acquaint yourself with the following list and use it as a guide when evaluating any policy:

- The policy should provide a daily nursing home benefit of at least *$100.* The range of daily benefits is generally $40 to $200.

- The waiting period before benefits begin should be no more than *20 days.* This is known as the *elimination period.*

- The maximum benefit period should be at least *four years* for one stay. If no time period is given, the dollar ceiling per benefit period should be at least 1,460 (365 days times 4) times the daily benefit. Ideally, the maximum benefit period for all stays should be *unlimited.*

- It should pay full benefits for skilled nursing facilities, intermediate care facilities and custodial care.

- If there is a rule requiring that you be in a hospital before entering the nursing home, *coverage should begin within 30 days after a hospital stay of three days or more.*

- It should pay *home care benefits.*

- Home health benefits should be paid *without* requiring a prior nursing home or hospital stay.

- It should have *waiver of premium,* which means that you need not pay premiums while you are in a hospital or nursing home. (You may have to pay extra for waiver of premium, but it should be available at least as an option.)

- It should be *guaranteed renewable for life.*

- The policy should specifically state that *Alzheimer's disease is covered.*

- The premium should stay *level for life.*

- The *Best's Insurance Reports Life/Health* rating of the company should be *A* or *A+*. (Best's is a service that, among other things, assesses the financial health of insurance companies.)

Some other points to watch out for:

- The insurance company may say your premium is level for life, but the contract may actually permit a rate increase if the company applies for one rate increase covering all the insured. Ask about this.

- Find out whether the company can decide whether you qualify for payments (usually on the basis of medical necessity). If so, what are your appeal rights?

- Find out how many nursing homes in your state the policy covers. Some policies pay only for selected homes.

- Find out whether nursing home care caused by a preexisting condition is covered. It almost surely will not be covered in full. The question is, how inconvenient are the restrictions? (For example, a waiting period during which Medicare pays for nursing home care [remember—skilled nursing facility only], after which the policy picks it up, is not bad. A two-year exclusion is too long; nursing home stays last an average of 838 days, or 2.3 years.)

Finally, resign yourself to the fact that no policy currently offered has adequate inflation coverage. The Brookings Institution has estimated that private insurance will cover only 7 to 12 percent of nursing home expenses in the year 2018 and that, at best, no more than half of the elderly will buy nursing home coverage.

Financial planners advise that no one under 60 buy a nursing home policy unless it offers some definite way to cover cost increases due to inflation. For those over 60, policies should be bought only by those who have more than modest assets. The rest of us should rely on Medicaid for nursing home coverage.

Selecting a Nursing Home

You can begin the process of selecting a nursing home by eliminating those you know you don't want to use. Don't consider nursing homes that:

- Are too far away to allow visiting by relatives and friends

- Are too expensive

- Are not properly certified or licensed

- Do not offer the medical or other services needed

- Are unsuitable for some other reason such as being owned by a religious denomination with which you do not want to associate

You can find out whether or not a home is properly certified or licensed by contacting the agency that regulates nursing homes in your state.

On pages 176-181 we provide a checklist for use in reviewing up to four nursing homes at one time. We suggest that you photocopy it and refer to it as you review homes in your area.

When you examine the checklist closely, you will note that some of the questions are starred. These questions can be answered only by your own observations.

Remember that you don't necessarily have to answer every single question on this checklist. You should try very hard to answer the ones that are important to you. If you forget to ask something important during your visit, you can always call later and try to get the answer; however, if you find that you didn't observe something important, the only way to get the answer is to schedule another visit. Look over the checklist carefully before you end each interview to ensure you have asked all the relevant starred questions. Then look over the rest of the questions before you end your tour to ensure that you have seen everything you need to see to answer them. *We suggest that you don't rely on memory. Circle the answer to each question as you observe or ask it.*

NURSING HOME CHECKLIST

	NURSING HOMES			
	A:	B:	C:	D:
Outside				
1. Is the building neat and well maintained?	Y N	Y N	Y N	Y N
2. Does it appear fireproof? (Wood-framed buildings can be dangerous.)	Y N	Y N	Y N	Y N
3. Are the sidewalks clean and well maintained?	Y N	Y N	Y N	Y N
4. Do the sidewalks have wheelchair ramps?	Y N	Y N	Y N	Y N
5. Does the entrance have handrails and wheelchair ramps?	Y N	Y N	Y N	Y N
6. Is the home located within easy walking distance of public transportation?	Y N	Y N	Y N	Y N
7. Are the grounds spacious?	Y N	Y N	Y N	Y N
8. Are they well maintained?	Y N	Y N	Y N	Y N
9. Is there an area where patients can sit?	Y N	Y N	Y N	Y N
10. Do they sit outside (weather permitting) or otherwise use the outside area?	Y N	Y N	Y N	Y N
Inside				
11. Is the lobby clean and well furnished?	Y N	Y N	Y N	Y N
12. Do residents use the lobby?	Y N	Y N	Y N	Y N
13. Are the corridors well lighted and wide enough for two wheelchairs to pass easily?	Y N	Y N	Y N	Y N
14. Does there seem to be enough room in general for the residents?	Y N	Y N	Y N	Y N
15. Are emergency exits well marked?	Y N	Y N	Y N	Y N
16. Is there an emergency lighting system?	Y N	Y N	Y N	Y N
17. Is there an actively functioning safety committee?	Y N	Y N	Y N	Y N
18. Is fire-fighting equipment (such as fire extinguishers) prominent?	Y N	Y N	Y N	Y N
19. Are there sufficient smoke detectors?	Y N	Y N	Y N	Y N

	NURSING HOMES			
	A:	B:	C:	D:

Rooms

	A:	B:	C:	D:
1. Are the rooms neat and clean?	Y N	Y N	Y N	Y N
2. Is there sufficient light?	Y N	Y N	Y N	Y N
3. Are there curtains on the windows?	Y N	Y N	Y N	Y N
4. Do all the rooms open on a hallway?	Y N	Y N	Y N	Y N
5. Do residents hang their own pictures?	Y N	Y N	Y N	Y N
6. Is there sufficient closet space?	Y N	Y N	Y N	Y N
7. Does each resident have a sink and mirror?	Y N	Y N	Y N	Y N
8. Is there counter space for personal objects?	Y N	Y N	Y N	Y N
9. Is the room nicely furnished?	Y N	Y N	Y N	Y N
*10. Is the room air-conditioned?	Y N	Y N	Y N	Y N
*11. Do the rooms have individual thermostats?	Y N	Y N	Y N	Y N
*12. Is there an adjoining bathroom?	Y N	Y N	Y N	Y N
*13. Are the bathrooms shared by no more than four residents?	Y N	Y N	Y N	Y N
*14. Do residents have a choice between single and jointly shared rooms?	Y N	Y N	Y N	Y N
15. In general, do residents have enough personal space?	Y N	Y N	Y N	Y N
*16. Are procedures for changing roommates liberal and clearly spelled out?	Y N	Y N	Y N	Y N
*17. If the rooms have television sets, are they equipped with earphones?	Y N	Y N	Y N	Y N
18. Do the beds have bedspreads?	Y N	Y N	Y N	Y N
19. Are there grab bars on the toilet and bathtub?	Y N	Y N	Y N	Y N
20. Do the tubs have nonslip surfaces?	Y N	Y N	Y N	Y N
21. Do bathrooms and toilet areas have sufficient privacy?	Y N	Y N	Y N	Y N
22. Do the rooms have private telephones?	Y N	Y N	Y N	Y N

Personnel

	A:	B:	C:	D:
* 1. Does the home's administrator have a current license?	Y N	Y N	Y N	Y N
2. Was the administrator or his or her representative courteous to you?	Y N	Y N	Y N	Y N
3. Did he or she see you promptly?	Y N	Y N	Y N	Y N
4. Were the home's administrative policies well explained?	Y N	Y N	Y N	Y N
5. Was the administrator open to your questions?	Y N	Y N	Y N	Y N
* 6. Does the home employ:				
a. a physical therapist?	Y N	Y N	Y N	Y N
b. an occupational therapist?	Y N	Y N	Y N	Y N
c. a speech pathologist?	Y N	Y N	Y N	Y N

	NURSING HOMES			
	A:	B:	C:	D:
d. a dietitian?	Y N	Y N	Y N	Y N
e. a nurse practitioner?	Y N	Y N	Y N	Y N
* 7. Is the nursing supervisor an R.N.?	Y N	Y N	Y N	Y N
* 8. Are all the head nurses R.N.'s?	Y N	Y N	Y N	Y N
9. Do there seem to be enough nurses, nurse's aides and orderlies on duty?	Y N	Y N	Y N	Y N
10. Was the staff generally friendly toward you?	Y N	Y N	Y N	Y N
11. Were they neatly dressed?	Y N	Y N	Y N	Y N
12. Did the residents seem at ease with the staff?	Y N	Y N	Y N	Y N
13. Did the staff speak to the residents in respectful, noncondescending terms?	Y N	Y N	Y N	Y N
14. Did the staff seem to like the residents?	Y N	Y N	Y N	Y N
15. **Did the staff members generally have pleasant expressions on their faces?**	Y N	Y N	Y N	Y N

Medical/Nursing Care

	A:	B:	C:	D:
* 1. Is a physician on the premises for a fixed period of time each day?	Y N	Y N	Y N	Y N
* 2. Is a physician on call in case of emergency?	Y N	Y N	Y N	Y N
* 3. Is a registered nurse on duty during the day, seven days a week?	Y N	Y N	Y N	Y N
* 4. Is at least one R.N. or one L.P.N. on duty day and night?	Y N	Y N	Y N	Y N
* 5. Are dental services provided in the home itself?	Y N	Y N	Y N	Y N
* 6. Are there facilities outside of the residents' rooms for physical examinations?	Y N	Y N	Y N	Y N
* 7. May the resident select his or her own physician?	Y N	Y N	Y N	Y N
* 8. May the resident select his or her own hospital?	Y N	Y N	Y N	Y N
* 9. Does the home have a contract with an ambulance service?	Y N	Y N	Y N	Y N
*10. Does the home have access to a pharmacist who maintains records on each resident and reviews them when new medications are ordered?	Y N	Y N	Y N	Y N
*11. Is the family allowed to make alternative arrangements for purchasing prescription drugs?	Y N	Y N	Y N	Y N
*12. Are arrangements made for patients who wish to use alternative professional services such as podiatrists or chiropractors?	Y N	Y N	Y N	Y N
*13. Does the home make arrangements for private duty nurses when the family thinks one is required?	Y N	Y N	Y N	Y N
*14. Does the home have policies that severely restrict the use of physical restraints?	Y N	Y N	Y N	Y N
*15. Are the majority of the residents free of physical restraints?	Y N	Y N	Y N	Y N

	NURSING HOMES			
	A:	B:	C:	D:
16. Are the rooms and halls free of any smell of human excrement?	Y N	Y N	Y N	Y N
17. Are they free of the smell of heavy perfume?	Y N	Y N	Y N	Y N
18. Does each resident have a call button within easy reach?	Y N	Y N	Y N	Y N
19. Can it be turned off only at the patient's bed?	Y N	Y N	Y N	Y N
20. Are there call buttons in the bathrooms and bathing areas?	Y N	Y N	Y N	Y N
21. Does each resident have a water container and clean glass in his or her room?	Y N	Y N	Y N	Y N
22. Are the more inactive residents' fingernails trimmed, and are the men cleanly shaved?	Y N	Y N	Y N	Y N
*23. Does the home keep its own medical records?	Y N	Y N	Y N	Y N
*24. Does the resident (or resident's family) have access to them?	Y N	Y N	Y N	Y N

Recreational/Social Arrangements

	A:	B:	C:	D:
* 1. Does the home employ a full-time social director?	Y N	Y N	Y N	Y N
* 2. Are residents permitted to entertain visitors in their rooms?	Y N	Y N	Y N	Y N
* 3. Are visiting hours liberal?	Y N	Y N	Y N	Y N
* 4. Are residents given reasonable leeway in establishing when they go to bed?	Y N	Y N	Y N	Y N
* 5. Are members of the opposite sex permitted to visit one another in their rooms with the doors closed?	Y N	Y N	Y N	Y N
* 6. Is alcohol permitted in the home?	Y N	Y N	Y N	Y N
* 7. Are there no limitations on outgoing or incoming telephone calls?	Y N	Y N	Y N	Y N
* 8. Do the published rules and regulations seem reasonable to you?	Y N	Y N	Y N	Y N
* 9. Are children permitted to visit?	Y N	Y N	Y N	Y N
10. Is there a quiet, private place where residents can entertain visitors?	Y N	Y N	Y N	Y N
11. Does there seem to be a wide range of recreational activities?	Y N	Y N	Y N	Y N
*12. Are residents included in this planning in some formal way?	Y N	Y N	Y N	Y N
*13. Is there an actively functioning patient council?	Y N	Y N	Y N	Y N
14. Is there sufficient room for the residents to engage in recreational/social events?	Y N	Y N	Y N	Y N
15. Are calendars of such events posted in convenient places?	Y N	Y N	Y N	Y N
16. Did you observe a substantial number of patients engaging in recreational/social events?	Y N	Y N	Y N	Y N

	NURSING HOMES			
	A:	B:	C:	D:
17. Is there a newsletter for families of residents?	Y N	Y N	Y N	Y N
*18. Are religious services held on the premises?	Y N	Y N	Y N	Y N
*19. Are arrangements made to allow patients to attend outside religious services if they wish?	Y N	Y N	Y N	Y N
20. Is there a library with recent magazine issues and a good selection of books?	Y N	Y N	Y N	Y N
21. Does the home sponsor frequent outings for those residents who are able to go?	Y N	Y N	Y N	Y N
22. Is there a canteen?	Y N	Y N	Y N	Y N
23. Do patients appear to socialize with one another?	Y N	Y N	Y N	Y N
*24. Does the home have any special programs with area schools to bring young people in to interact with the resident?	Y N	Y N	Y N	Y N
*25. Does the home subscribe to (and provide you with a copy of) a liberal Patient Bill of Rights?	Y N	Y N	Y N	Y N
*26. Is there a formal health education program for residents?	Y N	Y N	Y N	Y N
*27. Does the home provide frequent continuing education courses for its staff?	Y N	Y N	Y N	Y N

Food

1. Are fresh fruits and vegetables served in season?	Y N	Y N	Y N	Y N
2. Does the home prepare meals from scratch rather than use frozen or prepackaged meals?	Y N	Y N	Y N	Y N
3. Do the residents have a choice in the selection of meals?	Y N	Y N	Y N	Y N
* 4. Are provisions for special diets made?	Y N	Y N	Y N	Y N
* 5. Is help available for residents requiring feeding assistance?	Y N	Y N	Y N	Y N
* 6. Is this help available both in the resident's room and in the dining area?	Y N	Y N	Y N	Y N
* 7. Are residents served in their rooms if they prefer?	Y N	Y N	Y N	Y N
* 8. Is there a reasonable amount of flexibility as to when residents can eat?	Y N	Y N	Y N	Y N
* 9. Are dining hours for the convenience of the residents rather than the staff?	Y N	Y N	Y N	Y N
10. Are residents given sufficient time to eat their meals?	Y N	Y N	Y N	Y N
11. Does the food appear appetizing to you?	Y N	Y N	Y N	Y N
*12. Can the kitchen accommodate special, nonmedically prescribed diets (e.g., for religious reasons)?	Y N	Y N	Y N	Y N
13. Is the kitchen basically clean by your standards?	Y N	Y N	Y N	Y N
14. Does the kitchen staff appear neat and clean?	Y N	Y N	Y N	Y N
15. Is the menu cycle adequately varied?	Y N	Y N	Y N	Y N

	NURSING HOMES			
	A:	B:	C:	D:
16. Does the meal being served match the one on the menu?	Y N	Y N	Y N	Y N
17. Are the food carts closed for sanitation purposes?	Y N	Y N	Y N	Y N
18. Does the kitchen have a dishwashing machine?	Y N	Y N	Y N	Y N
*19. Are snacks available between meals and at bedtime?	Y N	Y N	Y N	Y N
*20. Do residents have access to a refrigerator to store their snacks?	Y N	Y N	Y N	Y N
21. Is the dining area clean and attractive?	Y N	Y N	Y N	Y N
22. Are the tables convenient for wheelchair use?	Y N	Y N	Y N	Y N

After the Visit

After you have completed the checklist, it may appear as though you have found out everything there is to know about the homes you have just visited. There is more to choosing a nursing home, however, than just answering questions. Your overall impression of each home is as important as its different services. One of the chief purposes of answering all these questions is to get this overall impression. (It is possible to have answered "yes" to all the questions in a particular category and still have a negative overall impression.) Therefore, we suggest that you do the following as soon after your visit as possible:

- Find a quiet place where you can work.

- Review the questions and answers under each of the six categories in the checklist.

- Attempt to rate each of the six categories on a scale of 1 to 5:
    1 Completely unsatisfactory
    2 Poor
    3 Adequate (barely)
    4 Good (improvement possible)
    5 Excellent

- Using these individual ratings, try to come up with an overall rating for each nursing home. Try to answer the following question:

    Overall, how do you rate this facility as a potential choice of nursing home?
    1 Completely unsatisfactory
    2 Poor
    3 Adequate
    4 Good
    5 Excellent

There is no magical way to come up with this important rating. In the final analysis, you (possibly with input from the potential resident if he is able to provide it) must decide how to weigh the different categories. A single "1" on some categories might be enough to exclude a home from serious consideration for most people. For others the quality of the medical or nursing care provided, or even the recreational or social services provided, may completely overshadow all others.

- Finally, place all the ratings (individual and overall) in the Overall Ratings Chart on page 183. (You may prefer to write in the words instead of the number—for example, "Poor" instead of "2.")

Overall Rating: This chart should now enable you to choose the best home from among the ones you have visited. If it doesn't, go back to the original Nursing Home Checklist and compare the homes question by question. If this still doesn't resolve the issue, try this next strategy.

A Final Strategy

If you still find it difficult to decide among the homes you visited, examine the reason for the problem. Is it because none is really suitable and you have to choose among the least of several evils? If so, consider visiting some more homes, possibly making a more systematic effort to get recommendations from acquaintances and health professionals.

In the first strategy, you rated each home "unsatisfactory" to "excellent," or you may have used a scale from 1 to 5. If this did not produce one home that seemed to stand out from all the others, perhaps you should consider converting your responses into percentages. A score of 90 percent in a particular category, or 90 percent overall, may tell you more about a particular home than a rating of "adequate."

If you decide to convert your responses into percentages, use the chart "Overall Ratings by Percentage of Responses" on page 183 along with the following steps:

- Go back to the Nursing Home Checklist and for each category (taking each home separately) count the number of "yes" answers you have recorded. (For example, under Nursing Home A, in the category "Rooms," you have 12 "yes" answers). Place this number above the fraction bar in the appropriate cell in the Overall Ratings by Percentage of Responses Chart.

- Now count the total number of questions you answered (both "yes" and "no") in a particular category (for example, under Nursing Home A, in the category "Rooms," you answered 15 questions). Put this number below the fraction bar in the appropriate cell. Your numbers should look like this:

$$\frac{12}{15}$$

OVERALL RATINGS CHART

	NURSING HOMES			
	A:	B:	C:	D:
Name				
Address				
Telephone				
CHECKLIST CATEGORIES				
Building and grounds				
Rooms				
Personnel				
Medical/nursing care				
Recreational/social arrangements				
Food				
Overall Rating				

OVERALL RATINGS BY PERCENTAGE OF RESPONSES CHART

CHECKLIST CATEGORIES	NURSING HOMES			
	A:	B:	C:	D:
Building and grounds	___ ___%	___ ___%	___ ___%	___ ___%
Rooms	___ ___%	___ ___%	___ ___%	___ ___%
Personnel	___ ___%	___ ___%	___ ___%	___ ___%
Medical/nursing care	___ ___%	___ ___%	___ ___%	___ ___%
Recreational/social arrangements	___ ___%	___ ___%	___ ___%	___ ___%
Food	___ ___%	___ ___%	___ ___%	___ ___%
Overall Rating	___ ___%	___ ___%	___ ___%	___ ___%
	6	6	6	6

- At this point you have a fraction. You should now divide the bottom number into the top number. In our example, when you divide 15 into 12, you get 0.8, which is then converted into a percentage by moving the decimal point two places to the right (0.8 = 80., or 80 percent). Or you could multiply the decimal by 100 (0.8 × 100 = 80 percent).

- You have now calculated the percentage response to your answers in one particular category. Now do this for the remaining categories.

- After determining the percentages in the remaining categories (remember, there are six), you can determine the overall percentage rating of a particular home. To do this, simply add the percentages determined in all six categories and divide by six (e.g., percentages 75 + 80 + 70 + 90 + 85 + 80 = 480 ÷ 6 = 80 percent).

Dealing With Problems That Arise in Nursing Home Care

It is difficult for nursing home residents to be effective advocates for themselves. If they are on Medicaid, they may have surrendered all their assets to obtain funding for their nursing home stay and may, in effect, be trapped in the home. They do not complain, simply because they do not want to make a bad situation worse. The same applies, to a lesser degree, to just about everyone else. Even if they are economically able to move, there may be long waiting lists at the homes they want to move to.

On the other hand, some people have completely unrealistic expectations of nursing homes. No patient in a nursing home should expect the attention that a private duty nurse in a hospital can give. No nursing home can afford to routinely provide that much service. Even if the service is excellent, it may not be possible to accommodate all residents' wishes for particular services (such as bathing) when they want it. But there's a minimum below which no nursing home should fall.

- No resident should be allowed to remain in a soiled bed a moment longer than absolutely necessary.

- It is close to impossible to prevent all pressure sores, but they should be small in size and promptly treated by positioning the patient, special mattresses and attention by a doctor when needed.

- Food should be hot or cold as appropriate and of better-than-just-acceptable quality.

- Dehydration and malnutrition should *not* develop and should be promptly and vigorously treated if found.

- Medications should be given and given reasonably close to the prescribed schedule. Drug reactions should be noted in writing and reported to the doctor quickly.

The best way to make sure that a friend or relative is getting the kind of services she should is by visiting frequently and randomly. It is good to arrange visits so that promised events can be checked on. If a particular program is scheduled—such as a movie, exercise, a walk or a presentation by a visiting speaker—visit when it is scheduled and make sure that it happens. Keep in mind that some cancellations are unavoidable due to weather and such, but the general program the home promises should be carried out.

Typically, it is best to deal with problems by pointing them out, politely but firmly, to the appropriate person—the nurse, the administrator, the billing office. The approach of being firm but not antagonistic works best. Keep repeating, in a polite manner, the problem you see and the solution you want. Let's look at the following example:

You discover that your mother has not had her heart medication for three days. You contact the nurse and tell her this. Ask why the problem occurred. Listen carefully. (If the answer is, "She bad a drug reaction, so we called Dr. Fanyatz, who said to stop the drug," then the right thing, not the wrong thing, has probably been done.) Depending on the response, you may need to suggest that the doctor be called or that the medicine be obtained from a local pharmacy while the nursing home's pharmacy is awaiting its receipt and so on.

An important point to remember is this: Don't let the nursing home put the monkey on your back. You do not have to solve, or even sympathize with, their difficulties. In some situations, the proper answer to "What would you suggest?" is, "I don't have to suggest anything. You have to find a way to deliver the services you promised, even if the pharmacy order is late."

Finally, it is not useful to threaten to move the patient. Besides the antagonism this may create, it may carry no weight in some areas. Many nursing homes have waiting lists and are well aware of the difficulties that often occur with nursing home placement. If a move is clearly indicated, make the arrangements and carry them out.

Home Health Services

You may be able to stay out of a nursing home with the assistance of home health care. Home health care consists of the following services:

- Part-time or intermittent nursing care provided by or under the supervision of a registered professional nurse (R.N.)

- Physical, occupational or speech therapy

- Medical social services provided under the direction of a doctor

- Part-time or intermittent services of a home health aide

- Medical supplies (excluding drugs and biologicals) and durable medical equipment

- Services of interns or residents of a hospital if the home health agency is affiliated with or under the control of the hospital

Not covered under home health care are 24-hour nursing care, transportation, housekeeping services and services that are normally not covered if provided in a hospital.

To qualify for home health services, you must be one of the following:

- In need of intermittent skilled nursing care, physical therapy or speech therapy

- Confined to your home or to an institution that is not a skilled nursing facility or rehabilitation facility

- Under the care of a doctor who is a medical doctor, osteopath or a podiatrist who determines that you need home health care and sets up a care plan

- In need of occupational therapy *after* a period during which skilled nursing care, physical therapy or speech therapy was needed

You are entitled to an unlimited number of home visits as long as you need the service. The home health agency providing the services must be one that is Medicare-participating.

You can have home health care visits for up to 21 consecutive days. After this, a gap of at least one day must follow before home health care visits can be prescribed again.

It is important to understand that home care under Medicare is composed of some (not all) *medical* (not custodial or intermediate) services that will allow you to remain at home rather than in a nursing home. It is not a "total care package" such as the social HMO experiments tried to provide.

Paying for Services Medicare Doesn't Cover

What can you do if you need services beyond what Medicare can offer? Many home health agencies offer these. They may include services such as delivery of hot meals, homemaker assistance and companions. Your supplemental insurance may cover some of these services for a limited time. You will also find that the home health agency is almost always willing to bill Medicare for the Medicare-covered services and bill you for the remainder. You may find that the charge for noncovered services such as homemaker assistance is affordable.

Many home health agencies will help you assess your home to see if modifications will make it more suitable for home care. If what is needed falls under the category of durable medical equipment and a doctor prescribes it, Medicare pays 80 percent of the cost and you pay 20 percent. Many vendors of durable medical equipment can tell you what Medicare covers and what it doesn't. You can also check with your Social Security office.

Some Cautionary Notes About Home Care

First, when ordering medical equipment and having your home checked for suitability for home care, make sure there is a way for you to terminate the rental or return the item if it turns out that it is not covered by Medicare and you decide you cannot afford it. You may be stuck with large expenses otherwise.

Second—and we regret having to mention this—you should make sure your money and valuables are in a safe place that you control before the home health worker visits. You should treat a visit from the home health worker like any other instance in which a stranger enters your home. There have been many instances of theft. Even very reputable agencies cannot always stand behind the ethics of every person they hire. You should ask the home health agency about its policies in cases of theft. Are they insured for theft by employees? What do they require in the way of proof? Is it enough to prove that no one other than the home health agency worker was in your home?

Because of prejudices against older people, you may be told that a stolen item was not stolen and you simply forgot where you put it.

(Of course, you should make sure that the item *was* stolen before you report it.) If something is stolen, report it to the police, to the home health agency and to your insurance agent if you have homeowner's or renter's insurance.

Third, as with all services, complain (politely) if you are unsatisfied. Home health agencies cannot make up for all the burdens of being old and ill, but they should, at a minimum, provide the medical services that were prescribed and any services that you are paying for—and should provide them well. Complain to the authorities that regulate home health agencies in your state if your discussion with the home health agency does not produce good results.

In this chapter we review: What to do when the system doesn't work ▪ How to appeal decisions involving your doctor ▪ How to protect your assets ▪ What to look for when purchasing insurance ▪ How to clarify problems when Medicare rejects a claim ▪ When to request a refund from a doctor for a service that wasn't medically necessary ▪ When and how to use the appeal process ▪ How to protect your rights

---

8. If It Can Go Wrong, It Will

The purpose of this chapter is to provide troubleshooting advice for dealing with the various things that can go wrong with the Medicare program. Medicare is so complicated that there are literally hundreds of reasons why a particular bill might not be paid.

The number of people and agencies who have a hand somewhere in the process is enormous. They include Congress, the Health Care Financing Administration (HCFA), the various federal district courts, the Medicare carriers and intermediaries, your various doctors, the hospital utilization review committee (URC), your managed care plan, the peer review organizations (PROs), your employer's or former employer's health care insurer, the employer's review agent, home health agencies, nursing homes and suppliers of medical equipment. Every one of them can do something somewhere along the way that can result in non-coverage of a medical expense you thought would be covered. It's a safe bet that in the vast majority of cases, you won't be told about it until you're informed that the bill hasn't been paid. And not having bills paid is just part of what can go wrong.

This chapter covers the most common problems under the following headings:

- Eligibility and Enrollment

- Hospitals

- Nursing Homes and Home Care

- Insurance

- Getting Bills Paid and Filing Claims

- Appeals

- Coordination With Employers' Health Insurance and Retirement Plans

Most of the chapter is in question-and-answer format, but we depart from this when the information can best be presented in some other way. Most of the questions are ones that People's Medical Society members have asked us over the years.

Three Important Points, Again

We'd like to emphasize three points raised earlier in this book that are important enough to bear repeating:

- You are not responsible for any medical bill you could not reasonably have been expected to know was not covered. But you have to make the case that you did not know that the service or expense was not covered.

- Increasingly, rejections of claims and termination or denial of services under Medicare are being based on *medical necessity*. If payment is denied, you usually have nothing to worry about—see the later section on claims. For denials of admission to hospitals, inpatient surgery and notices of noncoverage of further hospital or nursing home stays, you should work closely with your doctor; after all, it's *your doctor's* medical judgment that is being questioned.

- It is vitally important to *keep records* of your dealings with Medicare. For requests for reconsideration of denials, appeals and the like, it is important to *keep copies* of correspondence. When the correspondence has to be sent by a certain date, we recommend that you send it *certified mail, return receipt requested* so that you will have proof of mailing and proof of receipt. This is inexpensive, and the window clerks at any post office can show you how to do it.

You should also remember to *ask questions* (if you have them) of your local Social Security office. If the people there don't know the answer, they can refer you to someone who does. Keep asking until you get an answer and until you're satisfied it's the right answer. Your local Social Security office *is* your Medicare office for many issues. You can always call them and receive help or be directed to the right place.

Eligibility and Enrollment

I've applied for Medicare and have been told that I'm ineligible. What should I do?

Find out exactly why you are ineligible. (If you filed an application, you should receive a letter telling you the reason.) If you do not meet one of the *categorical* requirements of the program—for example, you are not yet 65, are under 65 and not disabled or are an alien not yet admitted for permanent residence—you should try to alter your status. (There's no way to be 65 faster, but you can consult a lawyer who specializes in disability cases, apply for citizenship or alien resident status and—if you were found ineligible because you had not worked enough—check your earnings record.)

If you feel that a clear error has been made and that it is not being corrected, you can appeal the finding of ineligibility.

You should also check to see if you are entitled on the basis of someone else's earnings. See chapter 2, which offers several examples. You may be eligible as the wife, widow, divorced wife, husband, widower, divorced husband, child or parent of someone else.

When should I apply for Medicare?

To be safe, you should apply for both Part A (hospital insurance) and Part B (doctor insurance) three months before you turn 65. This will allow you time to gather the proofs of earnings, date of birth and so on that you need and to clean up any errors in your earnings record. It will also prevent increases in your Part B premium due to late enrollment. Medicare and Social Security have been changing their procedures on automatic enrollment, and they may change them again. *If you want Medicare, apply for it.* Call your Social Security office for forms and procedures.

It is *very important* to remember that if you do not have 40 quarters of coverage (are not "fully insured"), you may need to continue working until you have earned the required number of quarters. Another option is that you may be eligible on the earnings of someone who is qualified for Social Security. This is especially important to spouses who may qualify on each others' work record or spouses who are now divorced but were married to each other for at least 10 years.

I suspect my earnings record at Social Security is wrong. How do I check it?

Contact the Social Security Administration at 800-772-1213 and request a copy of Form 7004-SM, *Request for Earnings and Benefits Estimate Statement,* or see chapter 2 for a sample letter.

I applied on the basis of disability and have been turned down. I want to appeal. What can I do?

Realistically, you have to hire a lawyer. Disability law is complicated, is affected variously by different precedents in different judicial districts and changes constantly due to court decisions. Beware of lawyers who promise to get you disability benefits. No one can promise that; it depends on the facts of your case. Also be aware that the federal regulations governing disability limit the fees the attorney may charge you for representation before the Social Security Administration. The fee is limited to the smallest of the following:

- Twenty-five percent of past-due benefits

- The fee you and the attorney agreed on

- The fee set by the Social Security Administration

If the case goes to a federal court, the court may award a fee higher than any of the above, but the amount the Social Security Administration will pay out of past-due benefits awarded is limited to the smallest of the three amounts. You are responsible for any fees above that amount that are awarded by the court. The Social Security Administration does not pay any fees if you lose because in that case there are no past-due benefits from which to pay. In other words, you always have to pay the attorney, but the fee is paid from past-due benefits if you win.

Before paying for an attorney, contact any senior citizens' centers, Area Agencies on Aging and welfare rights projects listed in the phone book. No-cost or reduced-cost legal services may be available from them.

I now know that I am definitely not eligible for Medicare. What can I do?

Persons 65 years old and older who do not otherwise qualify for Medicare can purchase Medicare coverage just like private insurance. This is expensive (see chapter 2). If you purchase Medicare coverage, you may choose from the same Medicare+Choice options that are available to those who qualify for Medicare. You'll find the information in chapter 2 very helpful when it comes to comparing plans and the coverage provided. Use the worksheets to carefully evaluate your options before making your choice.

You are permitted to purchase Part B of Medicare (doctor insurance) if you are a resident of the United States, are 65 or older and are either a citizen or an alien lawfully admitted for permanent residence who has resided in the United States for the past five years. (It is under this rule that everyone enrolls in Part B.) If you are not eligible for Part A of Medicare, enrolling for Part B entitles you to purchase it. So you have to buy Part B to get Part A.

How do I apply?

The first step in applying for Medicare is to call your local Social Security office. These offices are commonly listed under the federal government section in the blue pages of your local phone directory. If you can't find a listing, call directory assistance and ask for any Social Security office. Calling any Social Security office will enable you to find out which one you should go to.

Call that office. Tell them that you want to apply for Medicare (and Social Security if you are not already receiving it). The Social Security Administration is making a determined effort to carry out as much business as possible over the phone. This is generally more efficient, and it saves you a visit to the Social Security office. At the same time, if you have trouble dealing with matters like this over the phone (if, for example, you have trouble hearing and don't have an amplified phone), you can insist on a face-to-face visit. (For more on this, see chapter 2.)

Whichever way you apply, the Social Security office representative will fill out most of the forms for you. This is done to ensure that the type of answers the Social Security Administration needs to make a decision are obtained on the forms involved. After the representative has filled out the forms, you should read them—and insist on the correction of any errors—before signing them. If you need special assistance, special help will be made available to you. You may have to go to another Social Security office to find the right person to help you. The representative at the first Social Security office you go to will give you instructions. If you think you will need special help, you should mention this when you first call.

The representative will ask you to bring certain documents when you come to the Social Security office; usually, these include the following:

- Proof of age such as your birth certificate or a hospital birth record

- Records of earnings such as W-2 forms (or tax returns for the self-employed) for the past two years

- Your Social Security card

If you are applying because you think you should be considered disabled, you will be asked to bring some documents relating to your medical problems. The Social Security office representative will tell you what they are.

Keep your originals. Keep your originals. Keep your originals. More on the application process can be found in chapter 2.

I've lost my Social Security card and don't think I can remember the number. What can I do?

You need not worry if you have lost your Social Security card. If you can remember the number, you can apply for a duplicate. If you can't remember the number, it is likely to be on other documents around your house such as payroll stubs, credit card bills and insurance policies. If all else fails, the Social Security office can access its computer system, which will retrieve your name or any that sound like it. This considerably narrows the search for your number.

Hospitals

I want to visit my sister in Canada this summer and have some surgery done while we are together so she can take care of me. Will Medicare pay for a hospital stay outside the United States?

No. People think that Medicare pays for care anywhere in the world. It doesn't. Only care in hospitals in the 50 states and the District of Columbia, Puerto Rico and the last two U.S. territories—Guam and the Virgin Islands—is paid for. Care you receive in Europe, Canada, Mexico and the rest of the world is not covered. The only exception is if you are in the United States but are close to the Canadian or Mexican border and in need of emergency care, and the nearest hospital is in Mexico or Canada. In these situations Medicare will pay for the services provided.

Please note that doctors' services outside the United States are covered only if they are provided during an inpatient hospitalization that is paid for under the circumstances described earlier. *No other doctors' services outside the United States are paid for by Medicare.*

I am worried that I will have to leave the hospital when my DRG runs out, even if I'm not well.

Don't be. It's illegal for the hospital even to suggest it. During the early days of the Diagnosis-Related Groups (DRG) system, there were a number of instances of abuse. Patients were told they had to leave the hospital because their "DRG has run out" or some similar phrasing. Discharging any patient who still needs hospital care because of financial considerations is a total violation of the hospital's contract with Medicare. The hospital has agreed to provide services to you as long as they are medically necessary.

Because of the abuses that were observed, the People's Medical Society and the American Association for Retired Persons joined forces to ask Medicare to require hospitals to "Mirandize" Medicare patients—similar to the way that persons being arrested are told of their constitutional rights. Medicare now requires *all* hospitals to provide Medicare beneficiaries with an *Important Message from Medicare* (see pages 152-153) upon admission for any inpatient hospital care.

To sum up: The only reasons that you can be discharged from a hospital under Medicare are *medical* ones. Even if Medicare is no longer paying, you should not be discharged for lack of ability to pay. The hospital's social service staff should explore your eligibility for Medicaid and see what alternative sources of care are available. You may qualify for the "medically needy" category of Medicare based on your medical bills and inability to pay.

What do I do if the hospital tells me that I have to leave because my DRG has run out?

As we've said, this is (1) untrue and (2) a violation of the hospital's contract with Medicare. You are entitled to hospital services as long as they are medically necessary. The hospital can always apply for additional payment.

We suggest that you, or someone helping you, first write down the name and job title of anyone who told you this. Then call the hospital administrator's office. Tell her that you are aware that the hospital will be paid the full DRG for your admission. Tell her that you are aware that she can apply for outlier payments. Ask her if the hospital has done so. Then tell her the only reason that you can be discharged is because you no longer need hospital care. Tell her that hospitals don't discharge people—doctors do. Ask which doctor made the determination that you no longer need hospital care. Write down all the answers you get. Then call the Office of the Inspector General at the Department of Health and Human Services at 800-447-8477. Say that you want to report a case of abuse of the Medicare program. He'll take it from there.

I want to have an operation in the hospital, and Medicare has denied me, saying that I have to have it done in an outpatient facility. What can I do?

You can appeal, even though there is generally no problem with outpatient surgery, and you may be at less risk than you would be in the hospital. Your proposed admission was turned down because the PRO, or the URC acting for the PRO, did not find it medically necessary. You can request a reconsideration of this decision, just as you can any other PRO decision. The procedure is given below. Please note that this is a generic procedure for the filing of requests for reconsideration and appeals. These are two different stages of the same process; we refer to them all as "appeals" except where that might be confusing.

How to Appeal (Request a Reconsideration of) a Peer Review Organization Decision: You can appeal the decision of the PRO by filing a request for reconsideration with the PRO itself at the address for the PRO shown on the notice you received, at any Social Security office or at a Railroad Retirement office if you are a Railroad Retirement beneficiary.

Your doctor and the hospital also have the right to file an appeal. They do *not* have the right that you have to an expedited reconsideration.

Time to File the Request for Reconsideration: You must file your request for reconsideration within 60 days of the date you received the Notice of Noncoverage. Unless you can prove otherwise, the notice is deemed to have been received by you five days after the date on it.

Request for Extension of Time to File: If you need more than 60 days to file your appeal, you can request more time at any Social Security office or Railroad Retirement office. You cannot file an extension request with an intermediary. You will be notified in writing of the time granted you.

"Good Cause" for Late Filing: Generally, you will be allowed to file late if there is what the PRO considers to be "good cause" for it. The regulations give examples such as serious illness, a death in the family, failure to receive information you had requested before the 60-day limit, a misunderstanding of what the PRO notice told you and so on.

Obtaining Information: Both you and your doctor have a right to see the information on which the PRO based its decision. You should ask for this when you file your request for reconsideration. You may add anything to the information that you or your doctor want.

Expedited Reconsideration and Time Limits: You can request that the PRO make an expedited review and reconsideration of the denial. How fast "expedited" has to be depends on the circumstances:

- Within three calendar days if you are still a patient in the hospital and you receive a Notice of Noncoverage

- Within three calendar days if the initial determination was a pre-admission denial of hospital care

- Within 10 calendar days if you are in a skilled nursing facility

- Within 30 calendar days if you are appealing a hospital's decision not to admit you because it believes your proposed stay will not be covered by Medicare and in every situation in which someone other than you files the appeal. Having expedited redetermination available is a very important reason for you to file the appeal and have the doctor or hospital submit information as part of an appeal

What to Include: Follow the instructions on the information you receive from the PRO, or request an appeal with just a letter. You should ask your doctor to provide medical documentation. The general issues you will be dealing with are the medical necessity of the service, whether Medicare covers it, whether you are entitled to it and whether the amount paid is what ought to have been paid. Medical necessity boils down to appropriate medical judgment. Your doctor will probably want to submit information regarding your condition, plus evidence from the medical literature indicating that what the PRO wants done is unwise.

Notices and Appeals: When the PRO provides you with its reconsideration decision, it must do so *in writing* and inform you of the following:

- The decision

- The reasons for it

- A statement of the effect the decision has on what Medicare will pay for or has paid for

- A statement of your appeal rights, with complete instructions for filing the appeal

When you receive a notice of a reconsideration decision that is not in your favor, consider whether you want to request a hearing. A hearing is more formal than a reconsideration, and it entitles you to appear before an administrative law judge. If you do request a hearing, it is wise to have a lawyer involved. A hearing can involve subpoenaing witnesses and other legal steps. It is less formal than a court case but far more formal than a request for reconsideration.

Only you, not your doctor or the hospital, have the right to request a hearing. The rules for filing a request for a hearing are exactly the same as for filing for reconsideration with the PRO—60 days, counted from five days after the date of the notice. You should file your request for a hearing on HCFA Form 501.1 unless the information you received with the Notice of Reconsideration tells you to do something else.

You may request a hearing only if the amount in dispute is $100 or more.

As we said in chapter 6, the first thing the administrative law judge will attempt to determine is whether the controversy involves at least $100. If the judge determines that the amount is less than $100, he will notify you and any other concerned parties that he has determined this and that you and concerned parties have 15 days to show why he is wrong. If no evidence is submitted within 15 days, the request for a hearing is dismissed. (You will not have to worry about this if you don't receive such a notice.)

You will be notified by the judge of the date of the hearing at least 10 days before it is scheduled.

If the judge's decision is unfavorable, you can appeal to the Social Security Appeals Council. Your attorney can tell you how to do this. The Appeals Council does not take all the appeals addressed to it. If $1,000 or more is at issue, you can appeal an Appeals Council decision (or the judge's decision if the Appeals Council refused a hearing) to the federal courts. This must be done within 60 days of the date of the Appeals Council determination or its decision not to hear your case.

If you receive a favorable determination, Medicare pays its usual amounts for the services rendered. If you do not receive a favorable determination, you pay.

My doctor wants to do my operation in the hospital, but the PRO says no. What can I do?

See the answer to the preceding question.

Nursing Homes and Home Care

I need to go to a nursing home, but I'm not sure Medicare will pay for it. How can I tell?

Medicare does not cover what we usually think of as "nursing home care." There are three levels of nursing home care:

- *Skilled nursing facilities* offer care delivered by registered and licensed practical nurses on the orders of attending physicians. They offer services such as oxygen therapy; intravenous and tube feedings; care of catheters and wound drains; and physical, occupational and speech therapy.

- *Intermediate care facilities* provide less intensive care than do skilled nursing facilities. Patients are generally more mobile, and rehabilitation therapies are stressed.

- *Custodial, or sheltered, care* is nonmedical. Residents do not require constant attention from nurses and aides but need assistance with one or more daily activities or no longer want to be bothered with keeping up a house. The social needs of residents are met in a secure environment free of as many anxieties as possible.

Medicare covers nursing home care at the skilled nursing facility level only. This coverage is intended for basically one situation: care that you need in order to recuperate, but care that is less intense than that provided in a hospital. Medicare covers the first 20 days in full. From the 21st day through the 100th, you are responsible for a daily copayment (see page 46). Medicare picks up any amount over the copayment for these days. Beginning on the 101st day, Medicare pays nothing, and you are responsible for all costs. You are once again eligible for another 100 days of skilled nursing facility care in the next benefit period.

There should be no question that I need a nursing home and that Medicare will pay for it. After all, I can't do for myself a lot of the things that I used to. That's a health problem, and Medicare covers those—correct?

Not really. Nursing home care is covered only for a short time, and only if it will improve physical or mental functioning to a degree that makes the nursing home stay *medically* "reasonable and necessary." Medical necessity is *the* key issue in payment for skilled nursing facility services. The skilled nursing facility regulations go to great lengths to define what is and is not skilled nursing facility care. The key is this: Care that is complex enough to require the services of a nurse or skilled rehabilitation personnel is covered; care that you could do yourself is not. But complications may require skilled-nursing-facility-level care, even for situations that would normally not be covered. Basically, skilled nursing facility care is rehabilitation; if your condition cannot be expected to improve as a result of skilled nursing facility care *and* you do not need observation by skilled personnel, your care will not be covered. Obviously, what your doctor writes in the chart makes a big difference in what gets covered. If you are worried about coverage of skilled nursing facility services, discuss this with your doctor.

Is there anything I can do to stay out of a nursing home?

Yes. There are many alternatives that may enable you to stay out, depending on your level of functioning and the exact services you may need. Use the Health Status Checklist in chapter 7 to assess your needs.

For those who are not bedridden, adult day care, home health care, homemaker services, sharing a home with other elderly people, Meals on Wheels, shopping services and adult foster care may be alternatives that prevent the need for nursing homes. For the availability of these services, you can check with your local Area Agency on Aging, the medical social services office of the hospital (if the person is in the hospital awaiting discharge) and the state department of social services.

Many are listed in the telephone book under the "Guide to Human Services" section.

What about home health care? What does Medicare cover?

Home health care consists of the following services:

- Part-time or intermittent nursing care provided by or under the supervision of a registered professional nurse (R.N.)

- Physical, occupational or speech therapy

- Medical social services provided under the direction of a doctor

- Part-time or intermittent services of a home health aide

- Medical supplies (excluding drugs and biologicals) and durable medical equipment

- Services of interns or residents of a hospital if the home health agency is affiliated with or under the control of the hospital.

Not covered under home health care are 24-hour nursing care, transportation, housekeeping services and services that are normally not covered if provided in a hospital.

To qualify for home health services, you must be one of the following:

- In need of intermittent skilled nursing care, physical therapy or speech therapy

- Confined to your home or to an institution that is not a skilled nursing facility or rehabilitation facility

- Under the care of a doctor who is a medical doctor, an osteopath or a podiatrist who determines that you need home health care and sets up a care plan

- In need of occupational therapy *after* a period during which skilled nursing care, physical therapy or speech therapy were needed

You are entitled to an unlimited number of home visits as long as you need the service. The home health agency providing the services must be one that is Medicare-participating. You can have home health care visits for up to 21 consecutive days. After this, a gap of at least one day must follow before home health care visits can be prescribed again.

It is important to understand that home care under Medicare is composed of some (not all) *medical* services that will allow you to remain at home, rather than in a nursing home, and these only. It is not a "total care package."

Are there some things I should watch out for in regard to home health care?

First, when ordering medical equipment and having your home checked for suitability for home care, make sure there is a way for you to terminate the rental or return the item if it turns out that it is not Medicare-covered and you decide you cannot afford it. You may be stuck with large expenses otherwise.

Second—and we regret having to mention this—you should make sure your money and valuables are in a safe place that you control before the home health worker visits. You should treat a visit from the home health worker like any other instance in which a stranger enters your home. There have been many instances of theft. Even very reputable agencies cannot always stand behind the ethics of every person they hire. You should ask the home health agency about its policies in cases of theft. Are they insured for theft by employees? What do they require in the way of proof? Is it enough to prove that no one other than the home health agency worker was in your home?

Because of prejudices against older people, you may be told that a stolen item was not stolen and you simply forgot where you put it. (Of course, you should make sure that the item was stolen before you report it.) If something is stolen, report it to the police, to the home health agency and to your insurance agent if you have homeowner's or renter's insurance.

Third, as with all services, complain (politely) if you are dissatisfied. Home health agencies cannot make up for all the burdens of being old and ill, but they should, at a minimum, provide the medical services that were prescribed and any services that you are paying for and provide them well. Complain to the authorities regulating home health agencies if your discussion with the agency does not produce good results.

I've considered every alternative to care in a nursing home that you listed in chapter 7, and I still find I need nursing home care. Medicare won't pay for it. What can I do?

The Medicaid program covers nursing home care. Medicaid is intended for the very poor who have nowhere else to turn, but not all of the very poor are covered. It is a state-run program that receives federal funds. States make most of the rules, and the trend in recent years has been to make Medicaid requirements more stringent. Because these strict requirements forced many couples into poverty, Congress enacted new rules designed to limit impoverishment of the at-home spouse. Under these rules, the at-home spouse retains certain assets for living expenses, and half of the assets help to pay for the nursing home care of the other spouse. In this situation Medicaid doesn't pay the entire cost of care, and the at-home spouse isn't driven into poverty.

Here are some provisions of the legislation:

- In any month in which a married person is in a nursing home, no income of the at-home spouse is to be considered available to the spouse in the nursing home.

- Income is considered the property of the person to whom it is paid. Income paid to both spouses is attributed 50 percent to each.

- The home, household goods and personal effects of both spouses are not counted in considering Medicaid eligibility.

- All assets other than these will be counted and divided in two. If the at-home spouse has less than $16,152, the spouse in the nursing home may transfer assets to him to make up to $16,152 available to the at-home spouse. (States may, at their option, raise this figure to any amount less than $80,760. The $16,152 amount is indexed to inflation.)

- The assets that remain in the name of the spouse in the nursing home are considered available to pay for his nursing home care. All assets in excess of $80,760 are attributed to the spouse in the nursing home and are considered available to pay for nursing home care.

- States must allow nursing home residents to retain certain sums for medical expenses not covered by Medicare or Medicaid before contributing to the expense of their nursing home care. The states may place "reasonable limits" on the amounts spent.

- States must allow the at-home spouse sufficient income from the other spouse to bring total household income of the at-home spouse to at least 150 percent of the federal poverty level for a two-person household. States are not required to allow more than $2,019 per month, except by court order or change in regulation.

The current regulations require that the assets and income of your spouse and your parents be considered in determining your eligibility for Medicaid with few exceptions. This is a very important point: Your spouse and parents do not *actually* have to give anything toward the cost of your care, but your *eligibility* is determined as though they do. The exact requirements, as well as the amount of assets and income you may retain while still remaining eligible, vary from state to state because of the latitude allowed by the federal government in setting some of the income and assets limits. Check the list of state Medicaid offices in appendix E to find out where to call to determine the exact eligibility requirements for your state.

You are *automatically* eligible for Medicaid if you are eligible for, or receiving, Supplemental Security Income payments for the aged, blind and disabled, but you must apply at a state welfare office. If you meet the requirements for Supplemental Security Income, there is little chance that you would have to give up additional income or assets to qualify for Medicaid.

If your income, less certain deductions and medical bills, is within certain (low) limits, you may be eligible for Medicaid as medically needy. You must "spend down" to pay medical bills to the point at which you are eligible; after that, Medicaid pays for all medical bills as long as you are eligible.

But I don't have the money to pay my medical bills *now.* You're telling me that I have to pay them all off in order to get Medicaid to pay for future ones?

No. This is a common misunderstanding. The requirements for the medically needy "spend down" is that you have *incurred* enough medical bills so that your income, less allowances and the medical bills, is less than the income limit for eligibility. Medicaid pays all of the bills—both current and future—if you meet this test, have assets under the asset limit and meet any other requirements such as age and residency that your particular state may impose.

I don't want to give up my home. Can't I transfer it and my other assets over the limit to my children and continue to keep it?

You can transfer your assets to someone other than your spouse (for example, a child) in order to become eligible for Medicaid, but you must have done so within the time frame and manner permitted in your state. In addition, provisions found in the Health Insurance Portability and Accountability Act of 1996 impose severe penalties on individuals who *knowingly and willfully* dispose of assets in order to qualify for

Medicaid. As we've said before, do not dispose of any assets until you discuss your situation with a qualified attorney.

How do I apply for Medicaid?

Medicaid applications are taken at welfare offices, but many states also take them at senior citizens' centers, agencies on aging and other locations. Call the Medicaid office for your state (listed in appendix E) to find out where you can apply in your area. When you call the office in your area, find out what you need to bring with you for the application process.

Generally, you should bring proof of age, financial status and any disability you may have. The proof of financial status should include bank statements for checking and savings accounts, rent or mortgage payment receipts, loan papers for your car or the title to it, any documents relating to stock or bond ownership, and check stubs for any regular payments you receive. You should also have the amount of your Social Security check if you are currently receiving Social Security payments. You should always have your Social Security number. Bring your medical bills, or copies of them, from the past year.

How can I select a good nursing home?

You can begin the process of selecting a nursing home by eliminating those you know you don't want to use. Don't consider nursing homes that:

- Are too far away to allow visiting by relatives and friends

- Are too expensive

- Are not properly certified or licensed

- Do not offer the medical or other services needed

- Are unsuitable for some other reason such as being owned by a religious denomination with which you do not want to associate

Chapter 7 contains a checklist and several more suggestions for selecting a nursing home.

Now that I'm in the nursing home, I'm shocked by the conditions. What can I do?

It is difficult for nursing home residents to be effective advocates for themselves. If they are on Medicaid, they may have surrendered all of their assets to obtain funding for their nursing home stay and may, in effect, be trapped in the home. They do not complain simply because they do not want to make a bad situation worse. The same applies, to a lesser degree, to just about everyone else. Even if they are economically able to move, there may be long waiting lists at the homes they want to move to.

On the other hand, some people have completely unrealistic expectations of nursing homes. No patient in a nursing home should expect the attention that a private duty nurse in a hospital can give. No nursing home can afford to routinely provide that much service. Even if the service is excellent, it may not be possible to accommodate all residents' wishes for particular services (such as bathing) when they want it.

But there's a minimum below which no nursing home should fall:

- No resident should be allowed to remain in a soiled bed a moment longer than absolutely necessary.

- It is close to impossible to prevent all pressure sores, but they should be small in size and promptly treated by positioning the patient, utilizing special mattresses and arranging for immediate attention by a doctor when needed.

- Food should be hot or cold as appropriate and of better-than-just-acceptable quality.

- Dehydration and malnutrition should *not* develop and should be promptly and vigorously treated if found.

- Medications should be given and given reasonably close to the prescribed schedule. Drug reactions should be noted in writing and reported to the doctor quickly.

The best way to make sure that a friend or relative is getting the kind of services he should is by visiting frequently and randomly. It is good to arrange visits so that promised events can be checked on. If a particular program is scheduled—such as a movie, exercise, walk or presentation by a visiting speaker—visit when it is scheduled and make sure that it happens. Keep in mind that some cancellations are unavoidable due to weather and such, but whatever general program the home promises should be carried out.

Typically, it is best to deal with problems by pointing them out, politely but firmly, to the appropriate person—the nurse, the administrator, the billing office. A firm but not antagonistic approach works best. Keep repeating, in a polite manner, the problem you see and the solution you want.

An important point to remember is this: Don't let the nursing home put the monkey on your back. You do not have to solve, or even sympathize with, their difficulties. In some situations the proper answer to "What would you suggest?" is, "I don't have to suggest anything. You have to find a way to deliver the services you promised and are being paid for."

Finally, it is not useful to threaten to move the patient. Besides the antagonism this may create, it may carry no weight at all in some areas. Many nursing homes have waiting lists and are well aware of the difficulties that often occur with nursing home placement. If a move is clearly indicated, make the arrangements and carry them out.

Insurance

I want to buy insurance to supplement my Medicare. What should I look for?

We suggest that at a minimum you purchase a policy that covers all the deductibles and copayments for hospital and doctor bills. This means that you will have to pay only what Medicare does not reimburse the provider for, and it limits your expense to relatively minor items (with the exception of nursing home care). To protect yourself from this expense, the policy should also cover the skilled nursing facility copayment for days 21 through 100. You should also look for policies that cover physician charges in excess of the Medicare-approved charge. Policies that cover these expenses should pay at least 80 percent of the excess fee up to the full balance billing limits for nonparticipating doctors. This offers you further protection from large out-of-pocket expenses, which already cost Medicare beneficiaries billions of dollars each year.

Here are some insurance policy features to look for:

- Guaranteed renewability

- No more than a six-month exclusion for preexisting conditions

- No limitations to single diseases such as cancer

- Payment for services in full rather than a fixed amount

- No waiting periods for coverage

In chapter 4 we explain more about supplemental insurance and give you a means of comparing policies.

Getting Bills Paid and Filing Claims

How do I file a Medicare claim?

You don't! Thanks to a change in Medicare regulations, physicians and medical suppliers must prepare and submit your Medicare claims for any Part B services you receive. More precisely:

- Your doctor or medical supply company file the claim even if neither of them accepts Medicare assignment.

- You cannot be charged extra for this service.

- You are responsible for paying the bill in full if the provider does not accept assignment. You will be reimbursed by Medicare.

- You should contact the Medicare carrier for your state if any provider refuses to prepare and submit your claim.

That's the long and short of filing a Medicare claim.

My doctor filled out my claim form, and I filed a claim with my supplemental carrier, yet here I sit with a pile of rejection notices in front of me and no check. What went wrong?

Well . . . what should be a simple, effective process offering maximum speed of payment for providers and minimum worry for beneficiaries doesn't always work that way. A large part of the problem is the number of hands spoiling the broth: your doctor, the Part B carrier, your supplemental insurance carrier, the PRO, Medicare itself and so on. Even with doctors and suppliers filing Part B claims for you, sometimes things can go wrong. But we do have suggestions for the situation you face. First, you need to find out why the claim was rejected. Check the message found on the Medicare Summary Notice (MSN) or the notice you received from your supplemental carrier. It may well be some variation of "claim already paid," "duplicate claim," "provider has not submitted claim," "no MSN submitted" or some such message. What happens is this:

- Your doctor completed the claim form as required by law but has not yet submitted it to the carrier. In this case you don't have an MSN to file with your supplemental insurer and, therefore, cannot recover your 20 percent copayment. Check with your doctor to find out when she is going to submit the claim.

- You paid in full for the service because your doctor does not accept assignment (she is, however, required to file the claim), but you never received your reimbursement from Medicare. The doctor has not submitted the claim to the carrier and legally doesn't need to for up to one year. However, Medicare has warned that doctors and suppliers who willfully and repeatedly fail to submit assigned or nonassigned claims within one year will be subject to sanctions.

- She's a doctor who does take assignment (and, therefore, bills Medicare directly for 80 percent of the approved charge), and her billing agency sent in a duplicate claim. You receive a rejection notice from Medicare because the claim has already been paid and your supplemental carrier has also paid the doctor. You were unaware that a duplicate claim had been submitted.

- Medicare has already paid its 80 percent of the approved fee on an assigned claim. You send Medicare a claim for the 20 percent copayment (which you must pay) instead of sending it to your Medicare supplemental insurer. Many carriers' computers often can't distinguish this situation from other duplicate claims, so you're told it's being rejected as duplicate rather than that you're filing a claim for something that you or your insurer must pay.

- You pay the doctor in full for the service you received because she does not accept assignment. The doctor files the Medicare claim, and you receive a check for 80 percent of the approved amount, as well as an MSN. You now submit a second claim to Medicare to collect for the difference between the approved amount and what you paid the doctor. You receive a rejection notice from Medicare stating that the claim has been paid. Your claim should have been sent to your supplemental carrier for the 20 percent copayment. Some supplemental insurance policies may also cover charges above the Medicare-approved amount.

Second, check for these other common reasons for claims rejection:

- Medicare paid for the maximum number of services you can have. For example, Part A of Medicare pays for home health visits for 21 consecutive days, but after that a gap of at least one day must elapse before more visits can be paid for.

- You sent Medicare a claim for a service that is covered under your Medicare supplemental policy *but* not under Medicare. Your Medicare supplemental insurer may maintain a help line (perhaps a toll-free number) that can help you determine where to file for what services. Also check your policy: It may provide a chart or a simple explanation of what should be filed with it and what with Medicare.

- The claim, or part of it, was not paid because the money was needed to meet the Part A or Part B deductible.

- For psychiatric services, you have already received the lifetime maximum number (190) of inpatient days.

But my claim was rejected because the PRO (or the carrier or the intermediary) found that it was not medically necessary. What should I do now?

You don't need to do anything unless the doctor (or some other Medicare provider) demands payment. As we've noted repeatedly: *You are not required to pay for any service that you could not reasonably have been expected to know was not covered by Medicare. The only circumstance in which you are required to pay is one in which you were informed that no Medicare payment would be made for the specific service and you agreed to have the service performed in spite of this.* That a service (a course of treatment, a single treatment, a hospital stay) was not medically necessary is a judgment that the PRO is in most cases making after the fact. Hence, you're not required to pay: You cannot reasonably have been expected to know that the PRO, three months down the line, would find that the service you received wasn't needed. Does the PRO function of judging medical necessity mean that what Medicare routinely pays for on one side of some state or county line will be routinely rejected on the other? The answer is yes. This is, however, the nature of medical peer review. Groups of doctors in one part of the country don't necessarily always agree with groups of doctors in another.

How do you make use of this protection? Remember that in the vast majority of cases, you owe the doctor nothing. (You will probably get at least one bill, if the doctor's billing service is at all efficient, before you get the MSN with the rejection notice.) If you get a bill, send the doctor a *copy* of the MSN (keep your original) together with the appropriate letter from those that follow.

Exactly how you make sure you don't have to pay, or get a refund if you have paid, is a bit complicated. The following letters cover all the situations you will encounter. The essence is this:

- For a participating or nonparticipating doctor whom you have not paid, you should pay nothing; just send the letter if the doctor bills you.

- For a participating or nonparticipating doctor whom you have paid, you are owed a refund within 30 days unless the doctor appeals, in which case he must pay the refund within 15 days after he receives the notice of the decision. If the decision is to pay him, you will receive a revised MSN.

For a Doctor Who Is a Medicare Participant or Who Accepted Assignment on the Rejected Claim, to Whom You *Have Not Paid* the 20 Percent Copayment

Your name
Your street address
Your city, state and ZIP code

The date *(Important!)*

Your doctor's name
His street address
His city, state and ZIP code

Dear Doctor *[insert your doctor's name]*:

I recently received your bill for $ *[insert amount]* for *[insert name of service such as "fulguration of warts," from bill or MSN]* rendered on *[insert date]*.

As you can see from the enclosed copy of my Medicare Summary Notice, Medicare has rejected this claim because the services were found not to be medically necessary. A notice to this effect should have been sent to you by Medicare.

I am sure that you always try to give me the best care you can and that doctors may differ from time to time. It is important that you know that I am not required to pay the 20 percent Medicare copayment under these circumstances. Depending on the circumstances, you may or may not be paid by Medicare for the other 80 percent of the Medicare-approved charge.

Please correct your records to show that I do not owe you anything for this service.

Thank you for your attention to this request.

Sincerely yours,
Your signature

For a Doctor Who Is a Medicare Participant or Who Accepted Assignment on the Rejected Claim, to Whom You *Have Paid* the 20 Percent Copayment *OR* For a Doctor Who Is Not a Medicare Participant or Who Did Not Accept Assignment on the Rejected Claim, to Whom You *Have Paid* the 20 Percent Copayment and Any Additional Amount

Use the letter on page 211, but change the fourth paragraph to read:

I would appreciate your refunding me the amount of $ *[insert amount]*, which I paid *[insert "by check number" and number if you paid by check, "by money order" and number if you paid by money order]* on *[insert date]*.

For a Doctor Who Is Not a Medicare Participant or Who Did Not Accept Assignment on the Rejected Claim, to Whom You *Have Not Paid* the 20 Percent Copayment and Any Additional Amount

Use the letter on page 211, but delete the fourth paragraph.

My claim wasn't rejected totally, but I got a notice that it was reduced because of a judgment of medical necessity. What does that mean?

Essentially, the situation is exactly the same as for a rejected claim, but the PRO found that some other procedure, logically part of what the doctor did, *was* medically justified. For example, a charge for a lengthy office visit was changed to a charge for a brief office visit, and the doctor was paid 80 percent of the approved charge for that. You can use letters similar to the ones cited. Samples with the appropriate changes follow.

For a Doctor Who Is a Medicare Participant or Who Accepted Assignment on the Reduced Claim, to Whom You *Have Not Paid* the 20 Percent Copayment

Your name
Your street address
Your city, state and ZIP code

The date *(Important!)*

Your doctor's name
His street address
His city, state and ZIP code

Dear Doctor *[insert your doctor's name]:*

I recently received your bill for $ *[insert amount]* for *[insert name of service such as "fulguration of warts," from bill or MSN]* rendered on *[insert date].*

As you can see from the enclosed copy of my Medicare Summary Notice, Medicare has reduced the charge for this claim because some of the services were found not to be medically necessary. A notice to this effect should have been sent to you by Medicare.

I am sure that you always try to give me the best care you can and that doctors may differ from time to time. It is important that you know that I am not required to pay more than the 20 percent Medicare copayment for the reduced claim under these circumstances.

Please correct your records to show that I do not owe you any more than this amount for this service.

Thank you for your attention to this request.

Sincerely yours,
Your signature

For a Doctor Who Is a Medicare Participant or Who Accepted Assignment on the Reduced Claim, to Whom You *Have Paid* the 20 Percent Copayment

Use the above letter, but change the third and fourth paragraphs to read:

I am sure that you always try to give me the best care you can and that doctors may differ from time to time. It is important that you know that I am not required to pay more than the 20 percent Medicare copayment for the reduced claim under these circumstances.

I would appreciate your refunding me the amount of $ *[insert amount],* which I paid *[insert "by check number" and number if you paid by check, "by money order" and number if you paid by money order]* on *[insert date].*

For a Doctor Who Is Not a Medicare Participant or Who Did Not Accept Assignment on the Reduced Claim, to Whom You *Have Not Paid* 20 Percent Copayment and Any Additional Amount

Use the letter on page 213, but change the third paragraph to read:

I am sure that you always try to give me the best care you can and that doctors may differ from time to time. It is important that you know that I am not required to pay more than the balance billing limit, less 80 percent of the Medicare-approved charge, under these circumstances.

For a Doctor Who Is Not a Medicare Participant or Who Did Not Accept Assignment on the Reduced Claim, to Whom You *Have Paid* the 20 Percent Copayment and Any Additional Amounts

Use the letter on page 213, but change the third and fourth paragraphs to read:

I am sure that you always try to give me the best care you can and that doctors may differ from time to time. It is important that you know that I am not required to pay more than the balance billing limit, less 80 percent of the Medicare-approved charge, under these circumstances.

I would appreciate your refunding me the amount of $ *[insert amount]*, which I paid *[insert "by check number" and number if you paid by check, "by money order" and number if you paid by money order]* on *[insert date]*.

My doctor says she doesn't have to correct the bill or pay the refund because she has a sign in her waiting room that says that Medicare may not cover some services. Is she right?

No. Medicare has specifically ruled that the display of such a sign does *not* excuse the doctor from correcting bills, reducing charges or paying refunds.

I've sent the letters you suggested, but my doctor is dunning me and I don't want my credit rating ruined. What should I do?

Review the situation to make sure that you are facing a claim that you don't have to pay. (See chapter 3, the section "When You Never Have to Pay"). If you are reasonably certain, ask for assistance from the Medicare carrier or intermediary. If you have asked for assistance and have received none, call the Office of the Inspector General at the Department of Health and Human Services at 800-447-8477.

Appeals

As a Medicare beneficiary, you are entitled to appeal decisions and claims made by hospitals and other Part A providers, PROs, intermediaries, managed care plans and Part B carriers. All of these groups provide you with at least one level of appeal—a request for reconsideration. Part B carriers also provide you with a second level—a hearing before a hearing officer. If you are still not satisfied after you have exhausted this appeals process, you may be able to request a hearing before an administrative law judge or even take your case to federal court.

There are basically five circumstances in which you will want to appeal. The first is when a hospital or other Part A provider determines that Medicare will not pay your claim. The second involves decisions made by PROs concerning services that you are receiving or have already received.

The third circumstance involves a preadmission decision made by a hospital or skilled nursing facility. The provider determines that you will not be admitted because Medicare will not cover the cost of your care because it is not medically necessary.

The fourth circumstance involves decisions relative to your continued stay in a hospital or the proper setting for a service that you need. In this case you are a patient, and the PRO, your managed care plan or a review body such as the hospital's URC determines that your stay is no longer medically necessary and determines that Medicare will no longer pay. Or you are requesting a determination on whether or not you can be admitted to the hospital for a procedure that can be done on an outpatient, or ambulatory, basis.

The fifth involves claims submitted for services which you have already received under Part A or Part B and Medicare denies payment.

We covered much of this material in chapter 6. Some of that information is repeated below so that you won't need to page back and forth.

Appealing Decisions Made by Hospitals and Other Part A Providers

I've received a notice from the hospital that it believes Medicare will not pay for my care. Is this the same thing as a PRO determination?

No. Remember: If you receive a Notice of Noncoverage from a hospital or other provider, it is not an official notification as defined by Medicare. Therefore, you cannot appeal to Medicare. Rather, you must ask the provider to request a decision from Medicare. Here is the procedure:

- Ask your provider to get an official determination from Medicare.

- The provider must file a claim with Medicare on your behalf.

- Medicare will then issue a Notice of Utilization (this is the official Medicare decision).

- Based on the decision by Medicare, you may either agree with the decision or file an appeal.

The notice explains why the provider believes Medicare will not approve the service or why Medicare will not pay for the service. You may file an appeal by following the instructions on the Notice of Utilization.

Appealing Decisions of Peer Review Organizations

The PRO denied my request to have my surgery performed as an inpatient. Do I have any recourse?

Yes. PROs make decisions about inpatient hospital care, skilled nursing facility care and services provided in ambulatory surgery centers, and these decisions may be appealed. The procedure we cite is *generic*. It applies to *all* actions by the PRO. Only the evidence submitted would differ. See pages 155-159 for information on how to appeal a PRO decision.

Appealing Preadmission Decisions Made by Hospitals

I've been told that the hospital won't approve my admission, and I've learned that it made this decision without consulting the PRO. Is this legal, and can I still appeal this decision?

Yes to both questions. If you receive a notice from a hospital that it has reason to believe that Medicare *will not* cover your stay, it may decide not to admit you. In this situation it has made this decision without consulting the PRO. However, if you and your doctor disagree, file an appeal with the PRO. Here are the steps:

- The hospital's decision is not an official determination, so you must ask the PRO.

- You have 30 calendar days from the date you receive the hospital's decision.

- You have three calendar days to request an expedited review which may be done in writing or by telephone.

- The PRO will review the hospital's decision and send you its determination.

- If the PRO agrees with you and your doctor, the hospital must admit you, and Medicare will pay for your care.

- If the PRO agrees with the hospital, then you may request a hearing.

*Appealing
Decisions Made
by Intermediaries
on Part A Claims*

Medicare intermediaries handle most of the decisions made relative to hospitals, skilled nursing facilities, hospice care, home health care and a few inpatient matters not handled by PROs. If you disagree with the intermediary's initial decision on your claim, you have the right to appeal.

When I was admitted to the hospital for a surgical procedure, I believed it was covered in full by Medicare. Then I received my MSN and discovered that the intermediary denied my claim. What should I do?

The first step is to request a reconsideration from the intermediary itself. Do this after you receive your Notice of Noncoverage, which will come either in the form of an MSN or a letter. In any case it must be in writing. It will explain the reason that something is being denied. A typical MSN is shown on pages 78-79.

Time to File the Request for Reconsideration: You must file your request for reconsideration within 60 days of the date you receive the Notice of Noncoverage. Unless you can prove otherwise, the notice is deemed to have been received by you five days after the date on it. (For example, the notice is dated January 5. You are deemed to have received it on January 10 unless you can prove you received it later. The last day you can file an appeal is March 10, the 60th day after the deemed receipt of the notice.)

Request for Extension of Time to File: If you need more than 60 days to file your appeal, you can request more time at any Social Security office or Railroad Retirement office. You cannot file an extension request with an intermediary. You will be notified in writing of the time granted you.

"Good Cause" for Late Filing: Generally, you will be allowed to file late if there is what the intermediary considers to be "good cause" for it. The regulations are very broad, and it is hard to see what exactly might be considered good cause. The regulations give examples such as serious illness, a death in the family, failure to receive information you had requested before the 60-day limit or a misunderstanding of what the intermediary notice told you.

Obtaining Information: Both you and your doctor have a right to see the information on which the intermediary based its decision. You should ask for this when you file your request for reconsideration. You may add to the information anything you or your doctor want to add.

What to Include: You should file your appeal using HCFA Form 2649. You can request an appeal with just a letter, but using the form ensures that you include everything that is needed. You should ask your doctor to provide medical documentation. It is important for both you and your doctor to focus on the issue at hand and not to editorialize. You will be dealing with the general issues of the medical necessity of the service, whether Medicare covers it, whether you are entitled to it and whether the amount paid is what ought to have been paid. Medical necessity issues boil down to appropriate medical judgment. Your doctor will probably want to submit information regarding your condition, plus evidence from the medical literature that indicates that what the intermediary wants is unwise.

Notices and Appeals: When the intermediary provides you with its reconsideration decision, it must do so *in writing* and inform you of the following:

- The decision

- The reasons for it

- A statement of the effect the decision has on what Medicare will pay for or has paid for

- A statement of your appeal rights, with complete instructions for filing the appeal

When you receive a notice of a reconsideration decision that is not in your favor, consider whether you want to request a hearing. A hearing is more formal than a reconsideration, and it entitles you to appear before an administrative law judge. If you do request a hearing, it is wise to have a lawyer involved. Hearings can involve subpoenaing witnesses and other legal steps. A hearing is less formal than a court case but far more formal than a request for reconsideration.

Only you, not your doctor or the hospital, have the right to request a hearing. The rules for filing a request for a hearing are exactly the same as for filing for reconsideration—60 days, counted from five days after the date of the notice. You should file your request for a hearing on HCFA Form 501.1 unless the information you received with the Notice of Reconsideration tells you to do something else.

You may request a hearing only if the amount in dispute is $100 or more.

The first thing the administrative law judge will attempt to determine is whether the controversy involves at least $100. If the judge determines that the amount is less than $100, he will notify you and any other concerned parties that he has determined this and that you and concerned parties have 15 days to show why he is wrong. If no evidence is submitted within 15 days, the request for a hearing is dismissed. (You will not have to worry about this if you don't receive such a notice.)

You will be notified by the judge of the date of the hearing at least 10 days before it is scheduled.

If the judge's decision is unfavorable, you can appeal to the Social Security Appeals Council. Your attorney can tell you how to do this. The Appeals Council does not take all the appeals addressed to it. If $1,000 or more is at issue, you can appeal an Appeals Council decision (or the judge's decision if the Appeals Council refused a hearing) to the federal courts. This must be done within 60 days of the date of the Appeals Council determination or its decision not to hear your case.

If you receive a favorable determination, Medicare pays its usual amounts for the services rendered. If you do not receive a favorable determination, you pay.

Appealing Decisions Made by Carriers on Part B Claims

You also have the right to appeal decisions involving services covered under Part B of Medicare. This may include the request for a service, payment for a service or the decision not to pay for a service. If you disagree with the decision made by the carrier, you may appeal—following the information printed on the MSN—and you must do so within the time frame listed.

My doctor told me the scan she ordered was covered under Medicare Part B. When I received my MSN, I learned that the claim had been denied. What should I do?

You need to file an appeal with your Part B carrier. Here is the procedure:

- You write to the carrier and ask for a reconsideration of the decision.

- You have six months from the date the decision was made (the expiration date is printed on the MSN).

- You can mail or hand deliver you request to the carrier or contact any Social Security office or the Railroad Retirement office if you are a Railroad Retirement beneficiary.

- The carrier will send you a notice advising you of its decision.

If you disagree with the carrier's reconsideration decision, you may request a hearing before the carrier's hearing officer. You have six months from the date of the carrier's decision to file your request for a hearing. Use HCFA Form 1965 or a letter to request your hearing. You will receive a decision from the carrier's hearing officer advising you of its decision.

If you disagree with the carrier's hearing officer, you may request a hearing before an administrative law judge if your claim involves at least $500. You have 60 days from the date you receive the carrier's decision to request a hearing.

The judge will notify you of his decision. If it's in your favor, Medicare will cover the service. If the decision is *not* in your favor, you may appeal to the Social Security Appeals Council; however, the Appeals Council does not take every case that is addressed to it. If $1,000 or more is at issue and you disagree with the decision made by the judge and Appeals Council, you can appeal to the federal courts.

Appealing Decisions Made by Managed Care Plans

I'm enrolled in a Medicare+Choice managed care plan. Do I have the same appeal rights as those beneficiaries in regular Medicare?

Yes. As a Medicare beneficiary in a Medicare+Choice managed care plan, you have the same appeals rights as someone in the original Medicare program. The only difference under the Medicare+Choice program is that the initial review is conducted by the plan itself rather than by a PRO, intermediary or carrier. You may appeal any decision your managed care plan makes relative to your care if you think:

- The managed care plan has not paid a bill.

- The managed care plan has not paid a bill in full.

- The managed care plan will not approve or give you the care you think it should.

- The managed care plan is stopping care that you believe you need.

Your plan makes an initial determination based on information supplied by you and your doctor. The plan must respond within 14 calendar days (or 72 hours if you or your doctor request an expedited determination). Medicare requires that all requests for treatment be decided "as expeditiously as the enrollee's health condition requires."

If your plan denies your request for an expedited review, it goes into the standard 14-calendar-day review cycle. When your plan issues its decision, it must do so in *writing* and inform you of the following:

- The reason for it

- Your right to either a standard or expedited reconsideration

- A description of both the standard and expedited review processes

- A description of the rest of the appeals process with complete instructions for filing your appeal

If you are dissatisfied with the initial determination made by your Medicare+Choice plan, you have the right to request a reconsideration. The request for reconsideration is the first step in the appeals process.

A standard reconsideration must be completed within 30 calendar days, and an expedited reconsideration must be done within 72 hours. The process for requesting an expedited reconsideration is outlined below.

72-Hour Expedited Appeals Process

- File an oral or written request for a 72-hour appeal with your plan. Specifically state that you want an "expedited appeal, fast appeal or 72-hour appeal."

- Include a statement indicating that you believe your health could be seriously harmed by waiting for the normal 30-calendar-day appeals process.

- To file your request orally, call your plan. The plan will document your request in writing.

- To file your request in writing, mail, hand deliver or fax your written request.

The managed care plan informs you of its decision within the time frame based upon the type of appeal you file. If the decision is not in your favor, the managed care plan automatically forwards your appeal to the Center for Health Dispute Resolution (CHDR).

The CHDR renders its decision within 30 calendar days or within 72 hours if you request an expedited reconsideration.

Should the decision still not be in your favor, you may request a hearing before an administrative law judge, go before the Appeals Council of the Social Security Administration or take your case to federal court.

Coordination With Employers' Health Insurance and Retirement Plans

Plans are so varied and changes so rapid that it is hard to give specific advice. For most people Medicare will be your primary payer and your retirement insurance your secondary payer.

Keep in mind that employer-provided health insurance for persons over 65 who continue to work is now the primary payer, with Medicare picking up the difference between what the plan doesn't pay and what Medicare does—*not* the difference between what the plan pays and what you are charged. Group health plans must offer you the same health insurance benefit under the same conditions offered to younger workers. Look carefully at the list of Medicare-covered items in chapter 3. If you think Medicare covers something that the employer plan does not cover (the most common example is likely to be skilled nursing facility services), make sure you file a claim with Medicare.

Also remember that many employer health plans are, in fact, health insurance policies purchased from a carrier for a group of employees and are regulated by the insurance department or equivalent body in your state. Contact the insurance department if you suspect you are not receiving fair treatment or the benefits to which you are entitled.

My employer provides me with medical coverage as a retirement benefit, and I'm also on Medicare. If I need a service, who pays first?

In this situation Medicare will pay first, and your employers' health plan is your supplemental insurance. Remember: If you reject your employers' group health plan, your employer cannot offer you supplemental coverage. Consider very carefully how best to maximize your Medicare benefits; otherwise, you may find yourself without adequate coverage.

Appendix A: Medicare Intermediaries and Carriers

Intermediaries and carriers are insurance companies or other organizations that process and pay Medicare claims submitted by hospitals and doctors. Intermediaries process claims submitted by hospitals and other Part A providers, while carriers process claims submitted by doctors and other Part B providers.

When a claim is paid on your behalf, you receive a Medicare Summary Notice from the intermediary or carrier. This notice also contains important information on how to contact the intermediary or carrier if you have questions about the claim. For your convenience, intermediaries and carriers handle most inquiries by telephone. You will find the telephone number, usually toll-free, printed on the Medicare Summary Notice. Should you need to submit additional material, you will be given a mailing address.

Note: Some intermediaries and carriers serve more than one state or part of a state. You will be notified which contractor handles your claims. Contracts for intermediaries and carriers change from time to time, and you will be notified when these changes occur. Some telephone numbers may have changed; if this is the case, consult directory assistance.

Alabama
Blue Cross & Blue Shield of Alabama
205-988-2244
800-292-8855

Alaska
Blue Cross & Blue Shield of
   North Dakota
800-444-4606

Arizona
Blue Cross & Blue Shield of
   North Dakota
800-444-4606

Arkansas
Arkansas Blue Cross & Blue Shield
501-378-2320
800-482-5525

California
Residents of Imperial, Los Angeles,
   Orange, San Diego, San Luis Obispo,
   Santa Barbara and Ventura
   counties, contact:
Transamerica Occidental Life
   Insurance Company
213-742-3996
800-675-2266

All other residents, contact:
National Heritage Insurance
   Company
530-743-1583
800-952-8627

Colorado
Blue Shield of North Dakota
303-831-2131
800-332-6681

Connecticut
United Health Care, Inc.
203-237-8592
800-982-6819

Delaware
Xact Medicare Services
800-444-4606

District of Columbia
Xact Medicare Services
800-444-4606

Florida
Blue Cross & Blue Shield of Florida
904-355-8899
800-333-7586

Georgia
Cahaba Government Benefits
    Administrators
912-921-3045
800-727-0827

Hawaii
Blue Cross & Blue Shield
808-524-1240
800-444-4606

Idaho
CIGNA Medicare
208-342-7763
800-627-2782

Illinois
Health Care Service Corporation
312-938-8000
800-642-6930

Indiana
AdminaStar Federal
317-842-4151
800-622-4792

Iowa
IASD Health Services Corporation
Blue Cross & Blue Shield of Iowa
515-245-4785
800-532-1285

Kansas
Blue Cross & Blue Shield of Kansas
800-432-3531
800-432-0216

Kentucky
AdminaStar Federal
502-425-6759
800-999-7608

Louisiana
Arkansas Blue Cross & Blue Shield
504-927-3490
800-462-9666

Maine
C & S Administrative Services
207-828-4300
800-492-0919

Maryland
Trail Blazer Enterprises
800-444-4606

Massachusetts
C & S Administrative Services
781-741-3300
800-882-1228

Michigan
Michigan Medicare Claims
Health Care Service Corporation
313-225-8200
800-482-4045
800-562-7802 (area code 906)

Minnesota
MetraHealth Insurance Company
612-884-7171
800-352-2762

Mississippi
United Health Care Insurance
601-956-0372
800-682-5417

Missouri
*Residents of Andrew, Atchison,
    Bates, Benton, Buchanan,
    Caldwell, Carroll, Cass, Clay,
    Clinton, Daviess, DeKalb, Gentry,
    Grundy, Harrison, Henry, Holt,
    Jackson, Johnson, Lafayette,
    Livingston, Mercer, Nodaway,
    Pettis, Platte, Ray, St. Claire,
    Saline, Vernon and Worth
    counties, contact:*
Blue Cross & Blue Shield of Kansas
816-561-0900
800-892-5900

All other residents, contact:
General American Life Insurance
    Company
314-843-8880
800-392-3070

Montana
Blue Cross & Blue Shield of Montana
406-444-8350
800-332-6146

Nebraska
Blue Cross & Blue Shield of Nebraska
800-633-1113

Nevada
Blue Cross & Blue Shield
800-444-4606

New Hampshire
National Heritage Insurance
    Company
800-447-1142

New Jersey
Xact Medicare Services
800-462-9306

New Mexico
Aetna Life Insurance Company
505-872-2551
800-423-2925

New York
*Residents of Bronx, Columbia,
    Delaware, Dutchess, Greene, Kings,
    Nassau, New York, Orange, Putnam,
    Richmond, Rockland, Suffolk,
    Sullivan, Ulster and Westchester
    counties, contact:*
Empire Blue Cross & Blue Shield
516-244-5100
800-442-8430

Residents of Queens County, contact:
Group Health
212-721-1770

All other residents, contact:
Blue Cross & Blue Shield of
    Western New York
800-252-6550

North Carolina
CIGNA Medicare
336-665-0348
800-672-3071

North Dakota
Blue Cross & Blue Shield of
    North Dakota
701-277-2363
800-633-1113

Ohio
Nationwide Mutual Insurance
    Company
614-249-7157
800-322-6681

Oklahoma
Aetna Life Insurance Company
405-848-7711
800-522-9079

Oregon
Blue Cross & Blue Shield
503-222-6831
800-444-4606

Pennsylvania
Xact Medicare Services
800-382-1274

Puerto Rico
Triple S, Inc.
787-749-4900
800-981-7015

Rhode Island
Blue Cross & Blue Shield of
    Rhode Island
401-861-2273
800-662-5170

South Carolina
Palmetto Government Benefits
    Administrators
803-788-3882
800-868-2522

South Dakota
Blue Shield of North Dakota
800-437-4762

Tennessee
CIGNA Medicare
615-244-5650
800-342-8900

Texas
Blue Cross & Blue Shield of Texas
214-235-3433
800-442-2620

Utah
Blue Shield of Utah
801-481-6196
800-426-3477

Vermont
National Heritage Insurance
    Company
800-447-1142

Virginia
*Residents of Arlington and Fairfax
    counties, contact:*
Xact Medicare Services
800-444-4606

All other residents, contact:
MetraHealth Insurance Company
540-985-3931
800-552-3423

Virgin Islands
Triple S, Inc.
800-474-7448

Washington
Blue Cross & Blue Shield
800-444-4606

West Virginia
Nationwide Mutual Insurance
    Company
614-249-7157
800-848-0106

Wisconsin
Wisconsin Physicians' Services
    Insurance Corporation
608-221-3330
800-944-0051

Wyoming
Blue Cross & Blue Shield of
    North Dakota
307-632-9381
800-442-2371

Appendix B: National Association of Insurance Commissioners Standard Medicare Supplemental Insurance Policies

NATIONAL ASSOCIATION OF INSURANCE COMMISSIONERS STANDARD MEDICARE SUPPLEMENTAL INSURANCE POLICIES**

BENEFITS ↓ PACKAGE PLANS →	A	B	C	D	E	F	G	H	I	J
Core Coverage										
Part A Copayment Days 61–90										
Part A Copayment Reserve Days 91–150										
Parts A & B Blood Deductible	•	•	•	•	•	•	•	•	•	•
Part B 20% Copayment										
365 Lifetime Hospital Days 100%										
Additional Coverage										
Part A Hospital Deductible		•	•	•	•	•	•	•	•	•
Part B Doctor Deductible			•			•				•
SNF Copayment Days 21–100			•	•	•	•	•	•	•	•
At-Home Recovery				•			•		•	•
Excess Doctor Charges						100%	80%		100%	100%
Foreign Travel (Emergency Care)			•	•	•	•	•	•	•	•
Prescription Drugs								Basic¹	Basic¹	Extend²
Preventive Services					•					•

¹Basic prescription plan includes: $250 deductible; 50% copayment; and $1,250 maximum benefit.
²Extended prescription plan includes: $250 deductible; 50% copayment; and $3,000 maximum benefit.

**Only policies meeting these standards may be sold as supplements to Medicare.

The chart on the opposite page lists the 10 standard Medicare supplemental insurance packages that have been designed by the National Association of Insurance Commissioners. These standard plans make it much easier to shop for supplemental insurance because you are able to compare like coverage and premiums.

The heart of these insurance plans is a core of basic coverage that must be included in all plans. This is labeled as Plan A and includes the Part A copayment for hospital days 91 to 150, Parts A and B blood deductible, Part B 20 percent copayment and additional hospital days beyond Medicare coverage.

The other nine plans, labeled B through J, contain the core coverage plus variations of coverage. Nine plans cover preventive health care services. Excess doctor charges above the Medicare-approved amounts are covered by plans F, G, I and J. Prescription drugs are covered by plans H, I and J.

In order to determine whether a particular service is included with a specific plan, read across the top of the chart until you find the plan. Read down the chart and note the coverage indicated by the black dots.

If you have any questions concerning a particular plan or insurance company, contact your state insurance commissioner's office.

Appendix C: Patients' Bill of Rights

As a Medicare beneficiary, you have certain guaranteed rights. These rights protect you when you receive health care; they assure you access to needed health care services; and they protect you against unethical practices. You have these rights whether you are in the original Medicare plan or a Medicare+Choice plan. Your rights include the following:

- The right to protection from discrimination in marketing and enrollment practices
- The right to information about what is covered and how much you have to pay
- The right to information about all treatment options available to you
- The right to receive emergency care
- The right to appeal decisions that deny or limit payment for medical care
- The right to know how your Medicare health plan pays its doctors
- The right to choose a women's health specialist
- The right, if you have a complex or serious medical condition, to receive a treatment plan that includes direct access to a specialist

The following information is taken from several pieces of legislation including the Patients' Bill of Rights Act, the Patient Access to Responsible Care Act and the Access to Emergency Services Act. The information falls into the following categories:

- Access to care
- Quality assurance
- Grievances and appeals procedures
- Protecting the doctor-patient relationship

Access to Care

Choice of plans: Legislation requires that managed care plans with a closed panel develop a limited point-of-service option.

Adequacy of provider network: Legislation requires that each plan have a sufficient number of providers to ensure that consumers receive services in a timely manner.

Specialty care: Legislation requires that plans permit direct access to specialists for consumers with special medical conditions.

Chronic care referrals: Legislation requires that plans address the special needs of consumers with chronic conditions and develop a process for accessing specialty care when required.

Women's protections: Legislation requires that plans permit direct access to ob-gyn services, guarantee a minimum length of stay for a mastectomy and provide access to breast reconstruction.

Children's protections: Legislation requires that plans provide direct access to pediatric specialists when necessary.

Continuity of care: Legislation requires that provisions be made for uninterrupted care should there be a change in plans or provider network status. This applies to pregnancy, terminal illnesses and institutionalization.

Emergency services: Legislation requires that consumers have direct access to emergency services without prior approval.

Clinical trials: Legislation requires that plans permit consumers with serious or life-threatening conditions to participate in clinical trials when no standard treatment is effective.

Drug formularies: Legislation requires that plans with formularies have a process for consumers to gain access to medications not on the formulary when medically needed.

Nondiscrimination: Legislation requires that plans not discriminate on the basis of genetic information, sexual orientation, race or disability.

Health plan information: Legislation requires that plans provide consumers with uniform information about the plans' policies and providers.

Confidentiality: Legislation requires that plans have appropriate safeguards to keep consumer records confidential.

Ombudsman: Legislation requires that each state establish a health ombudsman office to help consumers with appeals and grievances.

Quality Assurance

Quality assurance: Legislation requires that each plan have a quality assurance program to monitor the quality of care and make improvements when necessary.

Data collection: Legislation requires that plans collect uniform performance data and make this information available to consumers.

Advisory board: Legislation requires that plans establish a public/private advisory board to develop a set of quality standards.

Provider selection: Legislation requires that plans be nondiscriminatory when selecting providers.

Utilization review: Legislation requires that plans develop a fair utilization review program in conjunction with providers.

Grievances and Appeals Procedures

Internal grievances: Legislation requires that plans maintain an internal grievance process and address consumer concerns in a timely manner.

External appeals: Legislation requires that consumers have access to an external appeals process when the plan's internal mechanism has been unable to resolve the dispute.

Protecting the Doctor-Patient Relationship

Anti-gag clause: Legislation requires that consumers have the right to all information on treatment options. This prevents a plan from offering providers incentives for not treating consumers.

Provider due process: Legislation requires that plans follow procedures when issuing termination notices to providers.

Medical necessity: Legislation requires that plans make all treatment decisions in accordance with generally accepted principles and standards of professional medical practice.

Insurer liability: Legislation requires that the states review the laws that currently exempt health plans from any liability relative to treatment decisions.

Appendix D: State Peer Review Organizations (PROs)

Peer review organizations are groups of doctors and other health care professionals who are paid by Medicare to monitor the quality of care you receive. If you have questions about the quality of care you received from a hospital or doctor, you may file a complaint with the PRO for your state.

PROs do not answer questions about your bill or Medicare coverage. For Part A or Part B billing or coverage questions, contact the Part A intermediary or Part B carrier for your state. Some telephone numbers may have changed; if this is the case, consult directory assistance.

Alabama
Alabama Quality Assurance
   Foundation
205-970-1600
800-760-3540

Alaska
PRO-WEST
907-562-2252
800-445-6941

Arizona
Health Services Advisory Group
602-264-6382
800-359-9909
800-626-1577

Arkansas
Arkansas Foundation for
   Medical Care
501-649-8501
800-272-5528

California
California Medical Review
415-882-5800
800-841-1602

Colorado
Colorado Foundation for
   Medical Care
303-695-3300
800-727-7086

Connecticut
Connecticut Peer Review
   Organization
860-632-2008
800-553-7590

Delaware
West Virginia Medical Institute
302-655-3077
800-642-8686, Ext. 266

District of Columbia
Delmarva Foundation for
   Medical Care
410-822-0697
800-645-0011
800-492-5811 Maryland

Florida
Florida Medical Quality Assurance
813-354-9111
800-844-0795

Georgia
Georgia Medical Care Foundation
404-982-0411
800-282-2614

Hawaii
Mountain-Pacific Quality
   Health Foundation
406-443-4020
800-497-8232

Idaho
PRO-WEST
208-343-4617
800-445-6941

Illinois
Iowa Foundation for Medical Care
515-223-2900
800-647-8089

Indiana
Health Care Excel
812-234-1499
800-288-1499

Iowa
Iowa Foundation for Medical Care
515-223-2900
800-752-7014

Kansas
Kansas Foundation for Medical Care
913-273-2552
800-432-0407

Kentucky
Health Care Excel
502-339-7442
800-288-1499

Louisiana
Louisiana Health Care Review
504-926-6353
800-433-4958

Maine
Northeast Health Care
   Quality Foundation
603-749-1641
800-772-0151

Maryland
Delmarva Foundation for
   Medical Care
410-882-0697
800-492-5811
800-645-0011

Massachusetts
Massachusetts Peer Review
   Organization
617-890-0011
800-252-5533

Michigan
Michigan Peer Review
   Organization
313-459-0900
800-365-5899

Minnesota
Stratis Health
612-854-3306
800-444-3423

Mississippi
Mississippi Foundation for
   Medical Care
601-948-8894
800-844-0600

Missouri
Missouri Patient Care Review
   Foundation
573-893-7900
800-347-1016

Montana
Mountain-Pacific Quality
   Health Foundation
406-443-4020
800-497-8232

Nebraska
Iowa Foundation for Medical Care
515-233-2900
800-247-3004

Nevada
HealthInsight
702-826-1996
702-385-9933
800-748-6773

New Hampshire
Northeast Health Care Quality
   Foundation
603-749-1641
800-772-0151

New Jersey
Peer Organization of New Jersey
908-238-5570
800-624-4557

New Mexico
New Mexico Medical Review
   Association
505-842-6236
800-279-6824

New York
Island Peer Review Organization
516-326-7767
800-331-7767

North Carolina
Medical Review of North Carolina
919-851-2955
800-722-0468

North Dakota
North Dakota Health Care Review
701-852-4231
800-472-2902
888-472-2902

Ohio
Peer Review Systems
614-895-9900
800-837-0664
800-589-7337

Oklahoma
Oklahoma Foundation for
   Medical Quality
405-840-2891
800-522-3414

Oregon
Oregon Medical Professional
   Review Organization
503-279-0100
800-344-4354

Pennsylvania
Keystone Peer Review Organization
717-564-8288
800-322-1914

Puerto Rico
Quality Improvement Professional
   Research Organization
809-753-6705
809-753-6708

Rhode Island
Connecticut Peer Review
   Organization
860-632-2008
800-553-7590

South Carolina
Carolina Medical Review
803-731-8225
800-922-3089

South Dakota
South Dakota Foundation for
  Medical Care
605-336-3505
800-658-2285

Tennessee
Mid-South Foundation for
  Medical Care
901-682-0381
800-489-4633

Texas
Texas Medical Foundation
512-329-6610
800-725-8315

Utah
HealthInsight
801-487-2290
800-274-2290

Vermont
Northeast Health Care Quality
  Foundation
603-749-1641
800-772-0151

Virginia
Virginia Health Quality Center

Residents of Richmond, contact:
804-289-5397

All other residents, contact:
804-289-5320
800-545-3814

Virgin Islands
Virgin Islands Medical Institute
809-778-6470

Washington
PRO-WEST
206-364-9700
206-368-8272
800-445-6941

West Virginia
West Virginia Medical Institute
304-346-9864
800-642-8686, Ext. 266

Wisconsin
Meta Star
608-274-1940
800-362-2320

Wyoming
Mountain-Pacific Quality
  Health Foundation
406-443-4020
800-497-8232

Appendix E: State Medicaid Offices

Medicaid is a government insurance program that pays for some of the health care expenses of people with low incomes, regardless of their age. Each state operates its own Medicaid program under rules established by the federal government.

Applications for Medicaid are taken at local offices of your state health or welfare department. If you cannot find a local telephone number for your area, call the number listed below. You will be given the location of the local office. Some telephone numbers may have changed; if this is the case, consult directory assistance.

Alabama
Medicaid Office
800-362-1504

Alaska
Medicaid Office
907-561-2171

Arizona
Medicaid Office
800-654-8713

Arkansas
Medicaid Office
800-482-8988

California
Medicaid Office
800-952-5253

Colorado
Medicaid Office
800-221-3943

Connecticut
Medicaid Office
800-842-1508

Delaware
Medicaid Office
800-372-2022

District of Columbia
Medicaid Office
202-727-0735

Florida
Medicaid Office
888-419-3456

Georgia
Medicaid Office
800-282-4536

Hawaii
Medicaid Office
808-587-3521
800-894-5755 (Molokai and Lanai)

Idaho
Medicaid Office
800-926-2588

Illinois
Medicaid Office
800-252-8635

Indiana
Medicaid Office
800-433-0746

Iowa
Medicaid Office
800-338-9154

Kansas
Medicaid Office
800-766-9012

Kentucky
Medicaid Office
800-635-2570

Louisiana
Medicaid Office
504-342-3891

Maine
Medicaid Office
800-321-5557

Maryland
Medicaid Office
800-332-6347

Massachusetts
Medicaid Office
800-322-1448
800-408-1253

Michigan
Medicaid Office
800-642-3195

Minnesota
Medicaid Office
800-657-3672

Mississippi
Medicaid Office
800-421-2408

Missouri
Medicaid Office
800-392-1261

Montana
Medicaid Office
800-362-8312

Nebraska
Medicaid Office
800-642-6092

Nevada
Medicaid Office
800-992-0900

New Hampshire
Medicaid Office
800-852-3345

New Jersey
Medicaid Office
800-356-1561

New Mexico
Medicaid Office
800-432-6217

New York
Medicaid Office
800-206-8125

North Carolina
Medicaid Office
800-662-7030

North Dakota
Medicaid Office
800-755-2604

Ohio
Medicaid Office
800-324-8680

Oklahoma
Medicaid Office
800-522-0310

Oregon
Medicaid Office
800-273-0557

Pennsylvania
Medicaid Office
800-692-7462

Puerto Rico
Medicaid Office
809-765-1230

Rhode Island
Medicaid Office
800-346-1004

South Carolina
Medicaid Office
800-549-0820

South Dakota
Medicaid Office
605-773-3495

Tennessee
Medicaid Office
800-669-1851

Texas
Medicaid Office
800-448-3927

Utah
Medicaid Office
800-662-9651

Vermont
Medicaid Office
800-529-4060

Virginia
Medicaid Office
800-884-9730

Virgin Islands
Medicaid Office
809-774-4624

Washington
Medicaid Office
800-562-3022

West Virginia
Medicaid Office
800-688-5810

Wisconsin
Medicaid Office
800-362-3002

Wyoming
Medicaid Office
800-457-3659

Glossary

Adjusted average per capita cost (AAPCC): The estimated cost of providing services to Medicare beneficiaries in a particular county based on the historical costs of traditional fee-for-service Medicare. The Health Care Financing Administration pays managed care plans up to 95 percent of this amount to provide services to beneficiaries enrolled in the plan.

Administrative law judge: An official charged with making decisions in matters of administrative, as opposed to civil or criminal, law.

Advance directive: A written document stating how you want medical decisions made for you if you lose the ability to make decisions for yourself. The two most common advance directives are living wills and durable powers of attorney for health care.

Ambulatory surgery: A large, although limited, range of procedures using operative and anesthesia techniques that allow the patient to recuperate at home, rather than in the hospital, immediately following the operation.

American Association of Retired Persons (AARP): A service and lobbying group comprised of people age 50 or over that has the Medicare program among its concerns.

American Medical Association (AMA): The largest, although not the only, trade association of American doctors.

Anesthesiologist or **anesthetist:** A person who administers anesthetics for surgery and diagnostic procedures. An anesthesiologist is always a holder of an M.D. or D.O. degree; an anesthetist may be a nurse-anesthetist or an anesthesia technician.

Annual coordinated election period: A period of time—specifically October, November and December of each year—during which Medicare beneficiaries have the opportunity to select a Medicare+Choice plan for the next year.

Assignment: A process in which a Medicare beneficiary agrees to have Medicare's share of the cost of a service paid directly to a doctor or other provider, and the provider agrees to accept the Medicare-approved charge as payment in full. For most services, Medicare pays 80 percent of the cost, and the beneficiary pays 20 percent.

Automatic enrollment: A process whereby those persons who began receiving Social Security or Railroad Retirement benefits prior to their 65th birthday are automatically enrolled in Medicare Part A and Part B when they turn 65.

Balance billing: The practice of billing Medicare beneficiaries for the difference between the amount Medicare reimburses a provider and the amount the provider actually charges for services.

Balance billing limit: A Medicare regulation that limits the maximum fee that a nonparticipating physician may charge a Medicare beneficiary to 115 percent above the Medicare-approved amount. The physician is prohibited from collecting the difference or balance between his regular fee and the balance billing limit.

Balanced Budget Act of 1997 (BBA): The federal legislation that created the Medicare+Choice program and expanded the service options available to Medicare beneficiaries.

Benefit period: A method for measuring a beneficiary's use of services covered by Medicare. A benefit period begins the day the beneficiary is hospitalized or enters a skilled nursing facility. It ends after the beneficiary has been out of the hospital or facility for a period of 60 consecutive days. If the beneficiary requires additional facility care after the 60-day period, a new benefit period begins.

Benefits and premiums: A set of uniform benefits that must be offered to all Medicare beneficiaries in the service area of a managed care plan. Premiums and cost-sharing (deductibles and copayments) must also be the same for all beneficiaries enrolled in these plans. Benefits may not be reduced nor premiums increased if a beneficiary uses more services than other enrollees.

Carrier: A private organization, usually an insurance company, that has a contract with the Health Care Financing Administration to process claims under Part B (doctor insurance) of Medicare.

Catastrophic illness: Any unusually expensive or lengthy illness that greatly exceeds an individual's ability to pay.

Center for Health Dispute Resolution (CHDR): A private organization with a Medicare contract that reviews decisions made by managed care plans relative to treatment decisions. The CHDR becomes involved in disputes between beneficiaries and their managed care plans.

Congressional Budget Office: The agency of Congress that prepares analyses of various national budget alternatives and studies budget-related issues for Congress.

Consumer protections: The Medicare+Choice regulations that require that all beneficiaries in managed care plans have certain rights, including direct access to specialists, a well-defined appeals process and a requirement for the development of treatment plans for persons with special or complex medical needs.

Coordinated care plan: A managed care plan that is a health maintenance organization, health maintenance organization with a point-of-service option, preferred provider organization or a provider sponsored organization. Coordinated care plans manage the care the beneficiary receives and permit less freedom of choice than fee-for-service plans.

Copayment: The portion of the cost of care an insured person is required to pay, while the person's insurance plan usually, but not always, pays for the majority of the cost.

Cost-based plan: A managed care plan that has a contract with Medicare to provide services to beneficiaries enrolled in the plan. Medicare pays providers a monthly fee based on reasonable costs. The fee may be adjusted if a beneficiary should require more extensive care or if the cost of providing services increases.

Custodial care: A level of nonmedical care for people who do not require the constant services of nurses or aides; also called sheltered care. It is designed for people who are capable of independent living but who may require some assistance with personal care and homemaking services.

Custodial care facility: A facility that provides medical or nonmedical services (for example, assistance in the activities of daily living) that do not seek to cure, are provided during periods when the medical condition of the patient is not changing or do not require continued administration by medical personnel.

Deductible: The amount that an insured person must pay before an insurance plan pays for any portion of the cost of health care.

Department of Health and Human Services: The federal department charged generally with administration of national welfare programs.

Diagnosis-Related Groups (DRG) system: A method of paying hospitals based on the average cost of treating patients with statistically similar conditions.

Diagnostic workup: The process of testing and checking various hypotheses about possible conditions a patient may have when a diagnosis cannot be immediately established from symptoms, history or routine tests.

Dialysis: Use of a machine to remove waste products or toxins from the blood to assist or replace kidney function.

DRG: *See* Diagnosis-Related Groups (DRG) system.

Durable medical equipment: Medical equipment that is intended to be used repeatedly, usually by the patient or a caregiver, rather than being used once or a few times and discarded. Examples include wheelchairs, hospital beds and oxygen tanks.

Durable power of attorney: A delegation of some authority to another, which lasts until revoked.

Earnings record: The record of amounts earned by each individual for whom Social Security taxes were paid. Maintained by the Social Security Administration.

Elective surgery or **procedure:** An operation or procedure that, given the patient's diagnosis and condition, can be performed at any convenient time. Contrast this with an urgent procedure, which must be done very soon, and an emergency procedure, which must be done immediately.

End-stage renal disease: Kidney disease that is severe enough to require lifetime dialysis or a kidney transplant. Patients with end-stage renal disease are eligible for Medicare and may be eligible for Social Security payments if found disabled.

Executive departments: The various entities within the federal government that ultimately report to the President (as opposed to Congress or to the Supreme Court).

Expedited review: A review conducted by a managed care plan, a peer review organization or the Center for Health Dispute Resolution that must be completed within 72 hours of receiving a request from a Medicare beneficiary for medical services or continued hospitalization. Expedited reviews are an option when asking a beneficiary to wait the standard 14 calendar days could pose a health problem. *See also* Standard review.

Face sheet: The top document in a patient's hospital chart, which the doctor attests is correct as to conditions and procedures in order to obtain payment from Medicare under the Diagnosis-Related Groups system.

Federal judicial districts: Major divisions of the United States that are under the jurisdiction of a single federal appeals court. The federal district courts make laws that establish precedents that the Social Security Administration and Medicare must follow, but these precedents have binding force only within the judicial district unless Congress aligns laws with them or the Supreme Court makes them the law of the land by upholding them when an appeal from the federal district court decision is filed.

Fee-for-service system: The traditional health care payment system in which providers, including physicians and hospitals, are paid after they provide services to consumers.

General enrollment period: The time from January 1 to March 31 of each year, when anyone eligible for Part B (doctor insurance) of Medicare can enroll in it.

General medical/surgical floor: The area of a hospital in which patients who do not require special treatment are cared for.

HCFA: *See* Health Care Financing Administration (HCFA).

Health Care Financing Administration (HCFA): The part of the Department of Health and Human Services that operates Medicare and, together with the states, Medicaid.

Health maintenance organization (HMO): A managed care plan that combines the functions of insurer and provider of care, giving most necessary care for a prepaid fee and placing an emphasis on prevention and careful assessment of medical necessity.

HMO: *See* Health maintenance organization (HMO).

Home health agency: An agency approved by Medicare for the delivery of home health services to Medicare beneficiaries.

Home health care: Care rendered in a patient's residence by employees of a home health agency or other approved providers of home health care.

Hospital-based physician: A doctor who treats patients exclusively or almost exclusively in hospitals and so uses the hospital as her office, the place of primary contact with patients. Often the hospital bills for her services and pays her a salary.

Iatrogenesis: Causation of illness by a doctor in the course of treating another real or putative illness.

Immediate review: The three-day process of a PRO's reconsideration of its previous decision.

Immigration and naturalization records: Records maintained by or issued by the Departments of State and Interior that show that an alien has legally entered the United States or has become a citizen.

Individual enrollment period: The time, running from three months before one's 65th birthday to three months after, during which one can enroll in Part B (doctor insurance) of Medicare without a premium increase for delayed enrollment.

Initial election period: The period of time that begins three months prior to an individual's entitlement to Medicare during which a Medicare+Choice plan may be chosen.

Initial enrollment period: A seven-month period beginning three months before a person's 65th birthday during which that person can submit an application for Medicare Part A and Part B.

Inpatient: Someone admitted to a hospital for care; an adjective applying to care given in a hospital.

Inpatient hospital care: Care that is rendered in a hospital to someone who has been formally admitted and temporarily lives in the hospital while receiving treatment.

Intensive care unit: A part of a hospital in which people whose life support requires constant monitoring or who require close and constant observation are cared for.

Intermediary: A private organization, usually an insurance company, that has a contract with the Health Care Financing Administration to process claims under Part A (hospital insurance) of Medicare.

Intermediate care facility: An institution that provides less intensive care than skilled nursing facilities. Patients are generally more mobile, and rehabilitation therapies are stressed.

Living will: A document executed prior to or early in the course of an illness, expressing one's wishes in regard to medical treatment if one becomes unable to direct the course of it personally.

Managed care: A system of health care delivery that links payment with the delivery of health care services with the aim of giving people access to quality, cost-effective health care.

Managed care plan: A type of health care plan that utilizes the principles of managed care; examples include health maintenance organizations and preferred provider organizations.

Medicaid: A federal/state program, established by the Title XIX of the Social Security Act, that provides medical care to the poor.

Medically needy: Eligible for Medicaid, not because of absolute lack of income, but because income, less accumulated medical bills, is below state income limits for the Medicaid program.

Medical necessity: Thought to be required by the prevailing medical consensus. What is medically necessary in one period or one area may not be so in another.

Medical necessity determination: A formal judgment, usually made for purposes of insurance payment, that a treatment was or was not medically necessary.

Medical savings account (MSA): A health insurance plan with a high deductible. Medicare pays the premium for the insurance plan and also makes a deposit into a beneficiary's MSA. The beneficiary uses the MSA to pay for services until the deductible is met. After the deductible is met, the insurance plan pays for services that are received.

Medicare: A federal health insurance program for people 65 or older, people of any age with permanent kidney failure and certain disabled people that covers the cost of hospitalization, medical care and some related services. The Medicare program is administered by the Health Care Financing Administration.

Medicare-approved charge: The amount that Medicare has determined is appropriate for payment to a physician for a service, based on his and his colleagues' histories of charge. *See also* Usual, customary and reasonable reimbursement system.

Medicare+Choice: An expansion of the original Medicare program that includes managed care plans such as health maintenance organizations, health maintenance organizations with point-of-service options, preferred provider organizations, provider sponsored organizations, private fee-for-service plans and medical savings accounts.

Medicare-participating physician: A doctor who has agreed to accept assignment on all claims from all Medicare beneficiaries in return for certain incentives.

Medicare Summary Notice (MSN): A form sent to a Medicare beneficiary after a claim is paid, indicating what Medicare has paid for and why.

Medigap: An insurance policy sold as a supplement to Medicare, usually but not always having coverage of copayments and deductibles as its main features.

MSN: *See* Medicare Summary Notice (MSN).

Notarized affidavit: A document, signed in the presence of a notary public, in which an individual asserts, under penalty of perjury, that an assertion is true; an informal, written form of testimony.

Notice of Noncoverage: Notification to a Medicare beneficiary that hospitalization is no longer medically necessary and Medicare coverage will cease, after which a beneficiary may be liable for all charges if she does not leave the hospital. The notice must be in writing and must be issued by a proper authority—the person's doctor, the hospital or the peer review organization. Each notice of noncoverage must contain instructions on how to appeal the decision.

Office of Management and Budget: The agency of the executive branch of government that prepares the budget the president submits to Congress each year and supervises spending by government agencies during the year.

Outlier: A case that falls outside the statistical norms of the Diagnosis-Related Groups system, either in total cost or in days of hospitalization required. Medicare makes additional payments for outliers if the peer review organization approves.

Outpatient: A person who receives hospital care without being admitted to the hospital; an adjective used to describe such treatment.

Outpatient surgery: Surgery performed without admission to a hospital, even though the surgery may be performed in the hospital.

Outpatient treatment: Treatment at a hospital, or in a setting outside a hospital, that does not require admission or temporary residence at the hospital.

Part A: The part of Medicare that covers inpatient hospital care, skilled nursing home care, home health care, hospice care and blood services; also called hospital insurance. Part A also covers the cost of pharmaceuticals administered in the hospital but does not cover the cost of outpatient prescription medications.

Part B: The part of Medicare that covers the services of doctors provided on an inpatient or outpatient basis, surgical services and supplies, clinical laboratory services, home health care, hospital outpatient services and blood services; also called doctor insurance.

Participating physician agreement: An agreement a doctor signs with the Health Care Financing Administration to accept assignment on all Medicare claims and to follow certain procedures; renewed annually.

Patients' Bill of Rights: A formal set of principles that recognizes Medicare patients are entitled to direct access to specialists, information on the financial condition of private health plans, disclosure of quality outcomes, confidentiality of patient records and the right to appeal decisions made by a Medicare provider.

Peer review organization (PRO): A group of doctors who have contracts with the Health Care Financing Administration to evaluate the medical necessity of care rendered to Medicare beneficiaries under the Medicare program and to investigate the quality of care provided to Medicare beneficiaries.

People's Medical Society: A nonprofit national health care consumer advocacy organization.

Permanently and totally disabled: A term of art under the Social Security Act, applying to persons who meet the definition of disability and qualify for Social Security payments and Medicare on that basis.

Point-of-service (POS): A type of managed care plan that allows the covered person to choose to receive a service from a participating or a nonparticipating provider, with different benefit levels associated with the use of participating providers.

POS: *See* Point-of-service (POS).

PPO: *See* Preferred provider organization (PPO).

Preferred provider organization (PPO): A managed care plan with a large network of physicians, hospitals and other providers.

Primary care physicians: Physicians who, by training, preference or necessity, practice a very broad range of medical services for persons not in need of highly specialized medical services; usually cited as including general practitioners, family practitioners, internists, pediatricians and gynecologists who take care of both their patients' gynecologic and general medical needs.

Primary diagnosis: The chief medical reason for an encounter with a health care provider or admission to a hospital.

Private duty nursing: Care given by a nurse who is hired to care for one individual exclusively in a hospital or nursing home and is paid directly by the individual or his family.

Private fee-for-service plan (PFFSP): A Medicare+Choice plan in which the beneficiary selects a private indemnity-type insurance policy that decides how much to reimburse practitioners for services provided. Beneficiaries are responsible for charges above Medicare-approved amounts and possibly for any additional premiums above the Medicare payment.

PRO: *See* Peer review organization (PRO).

Procedure: A manipulation of the body to give a treatment or perform a test; more broadly, any distinct service a doctor renders to a patient. All distinct physician services have "procedure codes" in various payment schemes.

Prospective payment: Payment made before a service is rendered and accepted as payment in full by the provider; the opposite of fee-for-service payment.

Protocol: A written plan for caring for a particular condition, intended as a guideline to physicians and usually adopted by a medical institution such as a clinic, hospital or health maintenance organization.

Provider: A doctor or entity (home health agency, hospital) approved to give care to Medicare beneficiaries and to receive payment from Medicare.

Provider sponsored organization (PSO): A managed care plan owned by doctors and hospitals. These plans contract with consumers and businesses to provide medical services. PSOs may also contract with the Health Care Financing Administration to provide services to Medicare beneficiaries.

PSO: *See* Provider sponsored organization.

QMB: *See* Qualified Medicare beneficiary (QMB).

Qualified Medicare beneficiary (QMB): A Medicare beneficiary who qualifies for financial assistance based upon income and resources. Federal law requires state Medicaid programs to pay Medicare costs such as deductibles, copayments and Part B (doctor insurance) premiums for those who qualify. Information on the QMB program is available from any state welfare office.

Quarter of coverage: One-fourth of a calendar year, during which a person earns enough, in employment covered by Social Security, to have the quarter counted toward the number needed (usually 40) to ensure entitlement to Social Security and Medicare.

RBRVS: *See* Resource-Based Relative Value Scale (RBRVS).

Reconsideration: The first level of appeal after a managed care plan, peer review organization, intermediary or carrier issues an initial decision regarding a service or payment for a service.

Relative value unit: A numerical value such as 1.5 or 30.5 that is assigned to every service provided by a doctor and used to calculate the payment for that service. The components of a relative value unit are the work or skill required by the physician, the office practice expenses and the cost of malpractice insurance. The relative value unit is multiplied by a dollar amount to calculate the actual payment.

Resource-Based Relative Value Scale (RBRVS): A physician fee schedule that takes into account the skills and knowledge required to provide medical services. Each service provided by a physician is assigned a relative value unit based on work required, practice expenses and the cost of malpractice insurance. There is also an adjustment factor based on geographic location. The RBRVS replaces the usual, customary and reasonable reimbursement system.

Retrospective payment: Payment to a provider after care is given; fee-for-service payment.

Risk-based plan: A managed care plan that has a contract with Medicare to provide services to beneficiaries enrolled in the plan for a fixed monthly fee. Risk-based plans are responsible for providing all required services and are therefore "at risk" for any costs that exceed their monthly fee. The beneficiary may not be charged for any excess expenditures.

Risk pooling: The fundamental idea behind insurance. A large number of people with a low probability of high-cost events share the cost, reducing their individual risks to the amount of their insurance premium rather than the full cost of an event such as an accident or illness; the fundamental concept of insurance.

Secondary diagnosis: A condition that exists in addition to the one that is the chief reason for an encounter with a health care provider or admission to a hospital.

Skilled nursing facility: An institution that offers nursing services similar to those given in a hospital to aid recuperation of those who are seriously ill. Contrast with intermediate care and custodial care, which may meet some minor medical needs but are intended primarily to support elderly and disabled individuals in the tasks of daily living.

SLMB: *See* Specified Low-Income Medicare Beneficiary (SLMB).

Social health maintenance organization (SHMO): An experimental program that tries to provide for the medical and social needs of the elderly and disabled in one, prepaid package.

Social Security Administration: The part of the Department of Health and Human Services that operates the various programs funded under the Social Security Act and determines eligibility for Medicare.

Social Security office: Local offices of the Social Security Administration, found throughout the country, which take applications for Social Security and Medicare and handle processing of Medicare requests for reconsideration and appeals.

Special election period: A period of time during which beneficiaries enrolled in Medicare+Choice plans that cease to provide services are permitted to select another plan.

Special enrollment period: An eight-month period of time during which a person who is covered by an employer group health plan when first eligible for Medicare may be able to delay enrollment in Medicare Part B without a premium surcharge and without waiting for a general enrollment period. The group health plan must be based on current employment and cannot be for retired people. The special enrollment period begins when the person is no longer working and the group health coverage ends.

Specialist: A physician who has elected to practice, and usually has special training in, some branch of medicine other than primary care, such as surgery, or who has an exclusive focus in one area of primary care, such as allergy, gastroenterology and ear, nose and throat care. Especially in urban areas, specialists are expected to have certification (from specialty societies or boards) that they have had adequate training in the specialty.

Specified Low-Income Medicare Beneficiary (SLMB): A Medicare beneficiary who is not eligible for the Qualified Medicare Beneficiary program but may still be eligible for financial assistance. The SLMB program is designed for beneficiaries whose income is slightly higher than the national poverty level. The SLMB program pays the monthly Part B (doctor insurance) premium; however, it does not cover the deductible, copayments or services not covered by Medicare.

Standard review: A type of review conducted by a managed care plan when a beneficiary or doctor submits a request to provide a service which may or may not be medically necessary. A standard review must be completed within 14 calendar days. *See also* Expedited review.

Supplemental Security Income: A program that provides small stipends to the elderly, blind and disabled who for one reason or another are not eligible for other, more generous welfare programs.

Swing beds: Hospital beds approved by Medicare for use as hospital or skilled nursing facility beds, depending on demand.

Terminally ill: Having an illness that is expected to result in death.

URC: *See* Utilization review committee (URC).

Usual, customary and reasonable reimbursement system: A means of determining payments to doctors based on statistical profiles of their and their colleagues' history of charges.

Utilization review committee (URC): A group of doctors in a hospital who reviews lengths of hospital stays and treatments from the standpoint of medical necessity.

Index

A

AARP. *See* American Association of Retired Persons (AARP)

Abandonment, defined, 20

Adjusted average per capita cost (AAPCC), defined, 64, 239

Administrative law judge, defined, 39, 239

Advance directive, defined, 140, 239

Age requirements, Social Security vs. Medicare, 29, 35

AMA. *See* American Medical Association (AMA)

Ambulance services, services covered, 47, 90

Ambulatory services, services covered, 47

Ambulatory surgery, defined, 73, 239

American Association of Retired Persons (AARP), defined, 24, 239

American Medical Association (AMA), defined, 17, 239

Anesthesiologist, defined, 133, 239

Anesthetist, defined, 133, 239

Annual coordinated election period, defined, 34, 239

Appeals/reconsideration

hospital payments, intermediaries, 155, 159-162, 217-219

hospitalization

carriers, 162-163, 219-220

Medicare+Choice plans, 163-164, 220-222

hospitalization decisions, peer review organizations (PROs), 155-159, 196-199, 216-217

Assignment

defined, 20, 21, 111, 239

importance, 112-116

new incentives, 116-117

states in which physicians are required to accept, 20

Automatic enrollment, defined, 40, 239

B

Balance billing, defined, 75, 239

Balance billing limits, defined, 26, 239

Balanced Budget Act of 1997 (BBA), defined, 25, 240

BBA. *See* Balanced Budget Act of 1997 (BBA)

Benefit period, defined, 48, 77, 240

Benefits and premiums, defined, 65, 240

Bills, guidelines for dealing with Medicare, 76-77, 208-214

Biologicals

defined, 50

services covered, 50

Blood services, services covered, 46, 47, 48, 88, 94

C

Carriers

appeals/reconsideration with hospitalization, 162-163, 219-220

defined, 18, 240

guidelines for dealing with Medicare, 76-77

Medicare, contact information, 224-227

role in hospitalization, 144-145, 147

role in Medicare, 24-25

Catastrophic illness, defined, 240

Center for Health Dispute Resolution (CHDR), defined, 77, 240

Chiropractor, services covered, 90

Claims, guidelines for dealing with Medicare, 76-77, 208-214

Congressional Budget Office, defined, 22, 240

Consumer protections, defined, 151, 240

Coordinated care plan, defined, 25, 240

Copayment, defined, 44, 240

Cost-based plan, defined, 56, 240

Cost-sharing, defined, 80

Coverage. *See also* Services covered

defined, 44

Custodial care

defined, 19, 241

services covered, 19, 169, 199

Custodial care facility, defined, 85, 166, 241

Cyclosporine. *See* Immunosuppressive drugs

D

Deductible, defined, 45, 241

Dentist, services covered, 90, 98

Department of Health and Human Services, defined, 39, 241

Diabetes, products/services, services covered, 51

Diagnosis-Related Groups (DRG) system

defined, 19, 81, 241

hospitalization, 81-83, 141-142, 150, 195-196

Diagnostic tests, services covered, 47, 48

Diagnostic workup, defined, 82, 241

Dialysis, defined, 28, 241

Disability

Medicare application, appeal guidelines, 192

Medicare eligibility, 29, 32

Social Security eligibility, 37-39

Divorce, Medicare eligibility, 30

Doctors. *See* Physicians

DRG system. *See* Diagnosis-Related Groups (DRG) system

Drugs

immunosuppressive, services covered, 47, 50, 94

prescription, services covered, 98

services covered, 50

Durable medical equipment, defined, 48, 241

Durable power of attorney, defined, 137, 241